30 Yea

CW01625384

es

Love, Care and Relief

30 Years – 30 Stories

Told by Patients, their Families and the Team of Hospice Africa Uganda

Edited by Anne Lezak, Charles Akowa, and Agasha Doreen Birungi

HAU/IHPCA

First edition published in 2023 by
Hospice Africa Uganda Publications

An imprint of AESOP Publications
Martin Noble Editorial / AESOP
28a Abberbury Road, Oxford OX4 4ES, UK
www.aesopbooks.com

A catalogue record of this book is available from the British Library.

First edition 2023

i.

Cover designed by: Julia Berberan

ISBN: 978-1-914938-22-1

Contents

List of Illustrations

Preface and Acknowledgements

The community needs the dying to make it think of eternal issues and to make it listen and give to others.

Cicely Saunders[1]

The idea for this book came from Dr Eddie Mwebesa, Clinical and International Programmes Director at Hospice Africa Uganda. Dr Eddie also supported the individual writers throughout this exercise of love and caring.

The 30 stories herein represent 30 years of inspiring, challenging, and sometimes heartbreaking work on behalf of Ugandans with terminally ill cancers and other life-limiting, painful medical conditions.

These stories bring to life the vision that has undergirded Hospice Africa Uganda (HAU) since Dr Anne Merriman founded Hospice Africa in 1992 as the model for Hospice Africa Uganda in 1993:

'Palliative care for all in need in Africa'.

To realise this vision, the HAU mission brings peace to the suffering in Africa through providing and facilitating affordable and accessible palliative care in Uganda and other African countries.

We wish to thank the patients who generously allowed their stories – and in many cases photos of themselves – to be shared, along with the Hospice Africa Uganda team members who did

[1] Shirley du Boulay and Marianne Rankin, *Cicely Saunders: The Founder of the Modern Hospice Movement*, p. 109.

the hard work of writing down their recollections of some wrenching experiences, along with their journeys, while being the incredible caregivers they are. In a couple of instances, family members of patients wrote down their own memories of the difficult experience of having a family member with advanced cancer; they explained how much it meant to them, to have HAU clinicians treat their suffering family member and offer support to distraught relatives at a critical time.

Most of all, these stories are a tribute to the incredible dedication, skills, and determination of Dr Anne Merriman, HAU's founder. She arrived in Uganda three decades ago, driven by her faith and her dream of creating an African model of palliative care. Hospice Africa Uganda and the thousands of lives its work has touched are a direct result of Dr Anne's vision, commitment, hard work, and passion for relieving pain in people suffering throughout Uganda and Africa.

When Dr Eddie with Dr Doreen Agasha (CED) initially asked the palliative care teams of Hospice Africa Uganda to write their stories, they did not realise how much we were all to learn from them.

These inspiring stories are written by both dedicated palliative care Ugandan clinicians (mainly our nurses) and by relatives of patients they cared for. This book includes descriptions of actual patient cases along with a number of brief, yet telling stories, from Hospice Africa Uganda team members, including their personal history with Hospice Africa Uganda.

Each one is moving in its own way, as they invite you into the homes to see the needs, and how with open hearts and hospitality, we bring comfort and holistic care to patients and families during this special time before the end of life. African palliative care serves them mainly in their own homes, where most Africans wish to be with their family and loved ones, at this special time of life.[2]

This book brings you into the homes of the African patients we visit, so different from the developed world. It shows African palliative care at its best, which can be delivered affordably in low- and middle-income countries (LMICs), in spite of different cultural needs and low country and family economies. The difference we make, demands our own compassion, medical, spiritual and social/emotional skills, Our interactions with patients and their families, and even their neighbours, have enabled us to translate Dame Cicely Saunders vision into true African palliative care.

About Hospice Africa Uganda and Our Palliative Care Work

Hospice Africa Uganda was founded in 1993 primarily to provide patients with life-threatening cancers relief from pain and comfort in their own homes and to spread relief from suffering throughout Africa.

Our vision of 'Palliative care for all in need in Africa' still stands but it is moving too slowly in most countries. Even in Uganda, our model country in palliative care, we are only reaching 14% of those in need with 80% of our Districts having at least one palliative care nurse. We have trained over 10,000 carers at all levels in Africa, yet it is still regarded in the health fields as unnecessary when set beside curative services. Caring is not seen as a priority by the established health services. Success

---

[2] E. Kikule.

is measured as maintaining life, not bringing peace to those at the end of life. Hopefully, readers of this book will realise that we can change this approach and the suffering in the homes through palliative care, but it must be suitable to the place where it is practised.

Our home care has expanded to clinics at our Hospice sites, outreaches to provide patient care in hospitals, to bring patient care and teach health workers, community volunteers and relatives the elements of hands-on palliative care. HAU also offers roadside clinics, where we see patients, often outside or in the Hospice car, or under a mango or suitably shady tree. Patients come to the location at specified times to meet a team of nurses from HAU, outside the usual catchment area. They consult, are examined and given treatment. This approach is a godsend for patients who can't make the long trip to the clinic at Hospice; and the palliative care team can see a number of patients at one place without having to make separate visits to often hard to reach locations.

Our dedicated teams at the three sites have shown remarkable commitment to this work over the years. You will read their own stories from their lives in palliative care in this volume.

The HAU teams are dedicated to our ethos, which has grown from the Hospice spirit which was there from the start in 1993. We have been blessed with dedicated team members from then until now; they still amaze me as they go the extra mile, often teaching me something new that brings us all closer to the patients we love.

As a physician, I have worked in many specialities on three continents, but the one that brings me the greatest return is palliative care. It is not highly paid; indeed, our team members have been on 50 per cent salary cuts in recent years. Funding is much reduced due to Covid taking over funding from donors and the health care system being focused on Covid and neglecting other causes of dying.

Our patients have so many needs and show so much gratitude. Most have never had a visit from a medical care team before. To see a loved one able to communicate after the team brought relief from terrible pain brings joy and peace to the whole family. Our teams are the Good Samaritans of their areas, bringing specialized treatment and loving care to all they meet.

This is God's work, and we must never forget this. The spirituality of our patients and of all in our teams is kept in mind at our daily prayer at Hospice sites and discussed with every patient. Uganda is so different to Western countries. I have yet to meet a Ugandan at the end of life who does not believe in God and most of them seek for their health worker to discuss existential issues with them.

May those who read this book be moved by the need for us to bring peace to those suffering in every situation but particularly in Africa and other LMICs, where typically fewer than 50 per cent reach any form of health care and 95 per cent of cancer sufferers do not receive curative treatment.

We ask for your prayers, your financial support, and your volunteering. Many volunteers come and return home changed people. Many have said to us in wonder 'we cannot do in the UK, US or other richer countries, what you have achieved here'. Yes we need financial support but most of all we need love and compassion, and this comes from the heart.

Anne Merriman

Annie Lezak

30 Stories for 30 Years

The year 2023 marks 30 years for Hospice Africa Uganda and birthed the idea of writing a collection of 30 stories. Teams at all our three sites at Hospice Kampala, Mobile Hospice Mbarara and Little Hospice Hoima embarked on writing something for this great milestone. They also gathered stories from patients.

The result is a captivating and moving book, full of life and all of the powerful emotions that come with extending love during the challenges facing patients with serious and life-limiting medical conditions and their families. It tells of the joys that come with never giving up on patients whatever the prognosis of the disease they have. It tells of the passion in teaching others how to care, showing compassion, and demonstrating excellent medical skills and providing important emotional support at the same time. It tells of hearts that seek to know patients, beyond theories that seek to define patients' illnesses. This is a powerful book of compassion.

As you read this book, may you be moved to demonstrate more than the expertise of your profession in life but to also extend love and care. Caring is still so vital in the world today as it was when Jesus told the parable of the Good Samaritan. Let us care for one another till the very end. Let us make it possible for those caring for the terminally ill to play their part by supporting their work.

Thank you for choosing to read this book today.

Dr Agasha Doreen Birungi
Recent Chief Executive Director
Hospice Africa Uganda

1

Venturing into the Unknown Arena

Rose Kiwanuka
First Palliative Care Specialist Nurse in Uganda

In 1993, Hospice and palliative care was not known to the public, nor was it clearly understood by health care workers. To me it was a new concept, I had never heard of it during my practice, not even in the nursing training school. Yet it is a specialty that should be practised and taught by all health care workers to complete the art of caring.

How I Got to Know about This Specialist Care

As a young nurse, caring for patients on a ward that combined gynaecology and surgical cases, I met a doctor who was particular about pain, who I later learnt was Dr Anne Merriman. Her interaction with a patient in pain was different. Whenever she came to a patient in severe pain, after a short conversation, she would give them a tablet, then continue the conversation. In her interview with patients, she gave them time and encouraged them to explain in detail the nature of pain they were experiencing in their local language. With a patient's consent, their carer was also involved during pain management session. This doctor either sat on a chair or a patients' bed when talking; she asked particular questions about pain, examined and even asked them to touch exactly where they felt pain. She documented in detail the way patients described pain, the possible cause of that pain and made diagnoses. Medications were prescribed according to nature of pain. She educated the patient, a nurse, and the carer in how to take the medication in the home. In the hospital she asked nurses to give it by the clock.

After several visits on my ward and seeing the outcome of her management I felt like changing my nursing approach and doing as she was doing. The challenge was the system: taking time talking to one patient, especially as a nurse, I would be seen as a lazy nurse who wasted time on the ward. A good hard-working nurse was expected to do a procedure on a patient within two to five minutes except for heavy procedures like wound dressing or bed baths. Consultants, senior doctors, and senior nursing officers had no idea about the approach to pain management. Besides there were a lot of myths about use of morphine for pain control and negative talks about Hospice and palliative care.

My Impetus to Join Palliative Care

The negative talk about palliative care by the senior doctors and my colleagues did not stop my inner drive to join palliative care. The more they talked negatively about it the more I felt the urge to care for terminally ill patients. I was propelled by the pain relief, peace, and comfort patients got after care. I particularly remember a patient who was isolated from the main ward because of offensive vaginal discharge due to cancer of the cervix and constant groaning due to pain. Her pain was controlled within ten minutes when she was introduced to pain control medication (morphine). The following day, there was no bad odour keeping away people from her room. That was my turning point: I realized how simple things like metronidazole, which was in plenty on the ward, could restore the patients' dignity when used differently. One time, when I suggested during a ward round that metronidazole tablets could be used on smelly wounds, the consultant rubbished my suggestion and added that he was the consultant to decide and introduce any treatment on the ward. I realized there was no room for nurses' input in the care for patients but just to take order from the doctors. I felt I was in a wrong place.

Changing from Curative to Palliative Care Nursing

In April 1994, I told my colleagues that I was joining palliative care nursing. They told me that was career suicide, and it was going to take me nowhere. They reminded me that Hospice and palliative care is about caring for the dying. I would soon get burnt out and leave nursing. I had seen how the last days of a patient were peaceful when a patient and family had come to terms with dying and a patient was pain free. I had seen a patient say goodbye peacefully to relatives around her.

In palliative care I was empowered to identify patients with palliative care needs including pain, to assess and manage their symptoms. I was legally allowed to prescribe opioids for patients in pain after being accepted for a Nurse Diploma in Palliative Care from Hospice Africa Uganda. Morphine has been the best medication recommended for severe pain by WHO for many years. That was a big motivation. I now had an answer to patients who would call me because of pain. The scenario of avoiding patients in pain because I had nothing to offer was over. I had crossed the burden of seeing patients in pain and doing nothing even when I knew what to do. I wanted more nurses to join palliative care nursing so that they could help patients who die in pain either in hospital or at home.

A nurse prescribing medications, including opioids for palliative care patients was not easily accepted by consultants and senior doctors. I remember prescriptions I made for patients being cancelled on different occasions. Slowly they realized that palliative care nurses were knowledgeable in pain management and legally allowed to prescribe opioids. With time, some of them started consulting and referring patients in pain to palliative care nurses.

Palliative Care Was Accepted as a Course in the Nursing Schools

The Ministry of Education and Sports launched an Advanced Diploma in Palliative Care Nursing in 2019 and the Mulago School of Nursing, the first government nursing school, enrolled 15 students on their first course. Since then, it has continued to enrol nurses interested in palliative care nursing and are supported by a scholarship programme I started through a partnership with Centre for Hospice Care in Indiana USA and

Palliative Care Association of Uganda, with the aim of empowering more nurses with palliative care knowledge to handle the increasing number of patients with non-communicable diseases. I also wanted palliative care to spread to various districts of Uganda so that it could be available to all who need it. In 2023, the government of Uganda is sponsoring seven nurses to undertake Advanced Diploma in Palliative Care Nursing. It is now clear that palliative care is engraved in the education and health care system of Uganda.

Joining palliative care is no longer career suicide but career progression because there are diploma courses and degrees, including a Masters degree and a soon to come PhD.

Never fear to venture into the unknown, it could be an opportunity for the entire world.

2

The Great Gift of Dr Anne and the Hospice Team

John Stephen Kafeero

In 1992, when I was studying to become an accountant, I went to visit my mother, who I learned was sick. She had malaria and was feeling as if her left side was a little paralysed. I decided to bring her to town because at that time I was at campus and our grandmother (her mother) was staying in Kampala.

The following day, I took my mother to Mulago Hospital. At Mulago, the doctors told us that she had malaria but with breast cancer as well. We learned the terrible news that the cancer had spread to the brain and was the reason for the paralysis of the left side. We got home and asked Mom, who explained to us that she had felt uncomfortable in her breasts but it did not seem serious, so she had neglected it. She did not understand what cancer was at that time.

My elder brother and I met a specialist the following day, who counselled us. My elder brother by that time was in theological college and his wife was studying at the teacher training college. The specialist told us that our mother was in the final stage of cancer and there was nothing much they could do about it. He said the best they could do was to give painkillers and that day the painkiller they gave was Panadol (paracetamol). He asked us not to bother bringing her to hospital because it was not going to help, as she was not going to survive. He told us that she would only survive for three weeks. This was very painful to hear.

After this I went and shared the whole story with Mrs Mukasa, a nursing sister at Nsambya Hospital, whose daughter was a friend of mine on campus. She told me that there was a lady who was a doctor in the hospital with a heart to care for such people. That doctor was Anne Merriman.

I still remember where I met Dr Merriman; we sat on two chairs under a tree just next to where she was living. There I narrated the whole story to her and she told me that she was just starting a Hospice and palliative care programme. Dr Anne told me to return the following day. We were so grateful because we didn't know how we were going to handle the pain and we didn't know how to care for a person in my mother's terrible situation.

Dr Merriman had a Land Rover, and when I went to see her the following day, she drove with me to Kitetika to meet my mother. That's when my mother became one of the very first patients of Dr Anne's programme. Dr Anne promised to assign some people to take care of my mother. She said the most important issue was pain relief because of the pain that had started to crop up due to Mom's illness.

So that's how I met Dr Merriman; and surely God works in mysterious ways because I don't know what we would have done if it wasn't for her. From that day, Dr Merriman and those nurses continued to visit nearly every three days. They gave my mother morphine, talked to her, encouraged her, counselled her, and rejuvenated her spirit, which seemed to have been lost.

The doctor at Mulago had already sentenced my mother and told her she would die in three weeks and she didn't know what to do. She had no one to take care of her children and she was demoralized. That's when Dr Merriman and others on her team came in and became her counsellors. In fact, my mother used to call Dr Merriman her sister because of the way she cared for her. She would sit on Mom's bed, and they talked over all sorts of things. There were times when Mom would ask us to get out of the room so that she could share some personal information with Dr Merriman.

One time Dr Merriman even spent a night at home because it was quite late for her to leave. Such special moments stick on the mind. My mother grew very close to Dr Merriman and also with the nurses on her team. The way they cared for my mother was like sisters caring for each other, like someone intimately caring for someone they know personally. Their hearts were amazing, and they did everything for my mother. They bathed her, fed her, and administered the medicine. They usually moved from Nsambya to our home in Kitetika using Dr Merriman's Land Rover. Every time people saw that car, they would say 'Sarah's sister has come.' Neighbours thought of them as sisters despite the fact that Dr Merriman was a 'Mzungu' (white person), due to the care, the love and the joy she brought to my mother.

In fact, the last person my mother talked to before she died was Dr Merriman. I remember she came that very evening, to administer what would be one of the last doses of morphine. It was close to 7:00 pm; she said she had had a lot of engagements that made her reach my mother's home quite late. She held my mother's hands and they prayed; my mother told her how she was feeling so weak, but Dr Merriman encouraged her. We had cooked mashed Irish potatoes. I gave her a few spoons of the food and then, around 30 minutes before midnight, my mother passed on. I still remember the last words my mother spoke to Dr Merriman; she said, 'I may be sailing home soon, but please take care of my children.'

Hospice care and palliative care are a rare service we cannot do without. Care at a personal level, with a personal touch, where someone cares for a patient as if they are caring for their close relatives. That is what Dr Merriman and those nurses (I think I can only remember Rose) did for my mother. They spend time with patients, fed them, prayed with them, and administered the painkiller. What a way for someone to sail home when they do not have to succumb to terrible pain! Cancer pain is too much, and you can't bear it on your own; you need help, you need counselling, you need assurance, you need care, and that's what Hospice offered to my mom.

The doctor gave my mom three weeks to live but fortunately, she took another nine months under that care. Nine months is quite a long time. However, there was no pain because the medicines they gave her kept the pain at bay. My mother was able to talk. She committed her life to Jesus, she talked to others about Jesus, she shared with us what she wanted to do and the things she wanted us to be, she gave us courage. This time prepared our minds, our thoughts, and our actions for her coming death. It also helped prepare her and her mother (because she was staying with her mother at that time) for what was coming.

Hospice is a candle in darkness and hope for the hopeless. When people sentence you to death and someone gives you another chance to live, that's a great thing. Hospice also prepares you to sail home peacefully without being in pain.

Three of my other aunties have unfortunately died of cancer, and it was a very painful experience. Hospice administers morphine and other drugs; they are so effective that you can't tell that the patient is very sick. Those drugs reduce the pain, which, along with the caring touch that Hospice gives, makes all the difference. Hospice gives you time to prepare, for example to write a will, and those caring for you have time to be with you, on a pain-free journey. Hospice service is very necessary and very important, not only to the patients but also to those who are relatives and friends of the patient. That is what I saw for my mother. I am so grateful to Dr Merriman and the Hospice team; they ceased to be nurses but became like dear relatives to us.

I did not know until recently that HAU welcomes donations; otherwise, I would have done it sooner. I have now encouraged all my siblings to support HAU. As someone extended that hand for free, why shouldn't we also do the same for others through this organization? HAU supports so many patients with cancer. Patients come to Hospice and receive medicine that cannot be afforded by a majority in Uganda, yet they get it for free at HAU. Some can't even afford food for patients, and HAU provides this.

Their work is so much needed in Uganda and beyond. I know HAU is overburdened, especially at this time. I encourage everyone to come out and support HAU to provide the much-needed care to patients and their carers.

3

Remembrance from a Grateful Daughter

Mrs Florence Kezia Kyazike Ssempiira (1995–1996)

Julie Nanjuki

My mother, fondly called 'Aunt Kezia' by all who knew her, was one of the greatest gifts God gave to our family. Aunt Kezia was a wife to Mr Fredrick Ssempiira, mother to five boys and a girl and a very enterprising woman.

In 1994, during school holidays, we got concerned over our mother's frequent fevers. Being the caring husband that Dad was, he always ensured that our mother received medication to bring down the fever. These fevers were on and off; after recovery, there was an aftermath of lack of appetite and selective eating or even refusal to smell or eat certain foods such as beans, which caused a lot of gas in my mother's stomach.

After about a year the stomach issue escalated to heavy bleeding with lots of clotting. Mum associated it to the family planning she once used as advised by a few friends. However, after two to three concurrent painful episodes (leaving her extremely weak), it was evident that she needed more medical attention than she was getting. Mum was taken to a nearby clinic where the nurse in charge only gave painkillers and advised that she visit a more equipped hospital for a scan.

On arrival at Mengo Hospital, she was told to see the gynaecologist. Dr Mirembe carried out an impromptu check-up and scan on my mother. When the lab tests were returned, Dr Mirembe suggested emergency surgery for my mother. According to her explanation to my father, Mum had cysts that were posing a huge threat to her life. She also confirmed the home nurse's suspicion that Mum had stage C cervical cancer. Little did we know what was in store for us as a family. Only later did we learn that at this stage the cancer is usually irreversible.

This shocking and sad news was secretly kept between the doctor and my father. However, with the scheduled operation and hospital stay, we could not help but be anxious.

Mum was operated on at Mengo Hospital and was able to return home. The recovery was slow but noticeable and she resumed some of her usual duties. However, it was short lived as she began to complain of so much pain. She could hardly sleep at times. During one of her review visits, Dr Mirembe recommended that she start on the chemotherapy as soon as possible.

Our mother's failure to recover fully raised concern among my siblings. My elder brother, who was at the university, decided to take matters into his own hands. He managed to get Mum's medical forms during one of the hospital visits and, without disclosing that the patient was his own mother, consulted his roommate, who was in the medical field.

Dan's roommate explained clearly what the diagnosis meant. He predicted that it would be a miracle for this patient to live for more than five years. Dan only had the strength to disclose this to our eldest brother. The rest of us just hoped and prayed.

Our mother was weak, but she did manage to go to Mulago for her chemotherapy sessions. However, her deterioration came as a shock to the entire family. Soon she was too weak to make it to hospital and complained of severe pain. The costs that come along with the treatment were extreme.

At a certain point, I could tell that my father was overwhelmed and was only trying to keep his head high. He hardly slept in the night even as he tried to keep his worries about Mum as discreet as possible. We could hear Mum groan from excruciating pain. For her the days were long, and so were the nights. The most unbearable part was watching a mother, wife, and friend wail over the pain, even through medication.

Dr Mirembe then suggested private care that was offered by Hospice Uganda. My mother's dear friends from the Union club of Namirembe Cathedral who often visited backed her suggestion and said that we needed professional help with making the patient as comfortable as possible. Dad immediately contacted the Hospice Africa Uganda team. Only one day later, a team visited our home.

This is what I fondly remember about the Hospice Uganda team. They used to visit in a team of 4–6 people (several were nurses doing palliative care practicums). Home was usually quiet to ensure that the patient was able to rest. As soon as the Hospice team arrived, the mood totally changed to beyond jovial. Even amidst the foggy mood and difficult circumstances, they were the kind of people you would love to host, over and over again.

phasized that they were not visitors but friends
On entering the patient's room, they would lighten
phere with words of encouragement. You would think
ey were long-time acquaintances of the family.

Mum responded well, always asking us if her friends would come. She loved the visits and the counselling sessions.

They engaged my mother in a very friendly way and took over all the responsibility during that time. They would discuss the progress and thank everybody for the good work being done.

Importantly, the team introduced medication that really reduced the pain. The Hospice team directed my mother's caretaker and several of my older brothers to ensure the patient had the medication at the proper time to effectively reduce pain. The caregiving was much better too. The Hospice team recommended a diet plan and general handling of the patient. Mum remained weak but was glad that she was comfortable.

During her last days, my mother was exhausted both mentally and physically, but the team did not give up on her. They visited more often during those days, when seeing her bedridden was detestable to the family. At one point, when she was very weak, they briefed the family on what we should expect with her impending death.

On 2 October 1996, she told my older brothers who were present that she accepted the fact that there was no point of return and that her grip on life had weakened. Later that night she slipped away into glory. It was a peaceful transition.

To say that cancer is harsh is an understatement; death is inevitable but how we die really matters.

I am so grateful to Hospice Africa Uganda; the journey was a lot easier with you by our side. Thank you for standing with us and understanding this cruel journey. Thank you for not giving up on us. We are still in awe at your consistency and friendly spirit. Thank you so much. May the Almighty bless you.

4

Cancer of the Cervix and a Mother's Worries for her Family

Martha Rabwoni

'Mary' was put on the Hospice programme in 2015 with a diagnosis of cancer of the cervix.

She had co-habited with two men and had six children, one of whom died. Five of the children, aged 9 to 16, belonged to the second. Mary never had a formal education; she was a peasant farmer.

In May 2015 she developed a vaginal discharge which had a bad smell. She went to a private clinic and was told she had syphilis. She was treated for that for some time without much improvement. In October 2015 she went to Mbarara Regional Referral Hospital (MRRH) where a biopsy was taken and she was found to be with cancer of the cervix stage 2b. She did get the good news that she was HIV negative.

Mary was prepared for radiotherapy. She was very worried about her children, who were young and would be left while she was away. The mother was the sole person in charge of their welfare. Additionally, finding someone to go with her as a carer to Mulago was not easy. Her eldest was 26 and married, so she could not go with her.

Eventually Mary managed to get to Mulago. After the radiotherapy she was well enough to go back to her usual work but not as energetic as before her sickness. She had problems with her man who continued to drink too much and to demand sexual intercourse which was now uncomfortable.

We called Mary's husband and talked with him, but it was not very helpful due to too much drinking. He is a toilet digger which yields little money that can support the family compared to what Mary had been earning. Her remission did not last long; after six months all her problems returned, and Mary became very ill. She had only her children to care for her and they no longer went to school which was very distressing. Making matters worse, the family had little to eat due to the long drought, which is nationwide problem, but made worse because Mary could do little work in her gardens.

Mary was a devoted Catholic and after a session of counselling, we suggested that maybe the priest could be persuaded to talk to the husband about supporting Mary and her children in this difficult time and she agreed. It did not work well because he kept avoiding the priest whenever he would come home.

Mary then developed rectal vaginal fistula and was completely bedridden. She and her two daughters who were helping her continually worried about how the family would manage when she was no longer there.

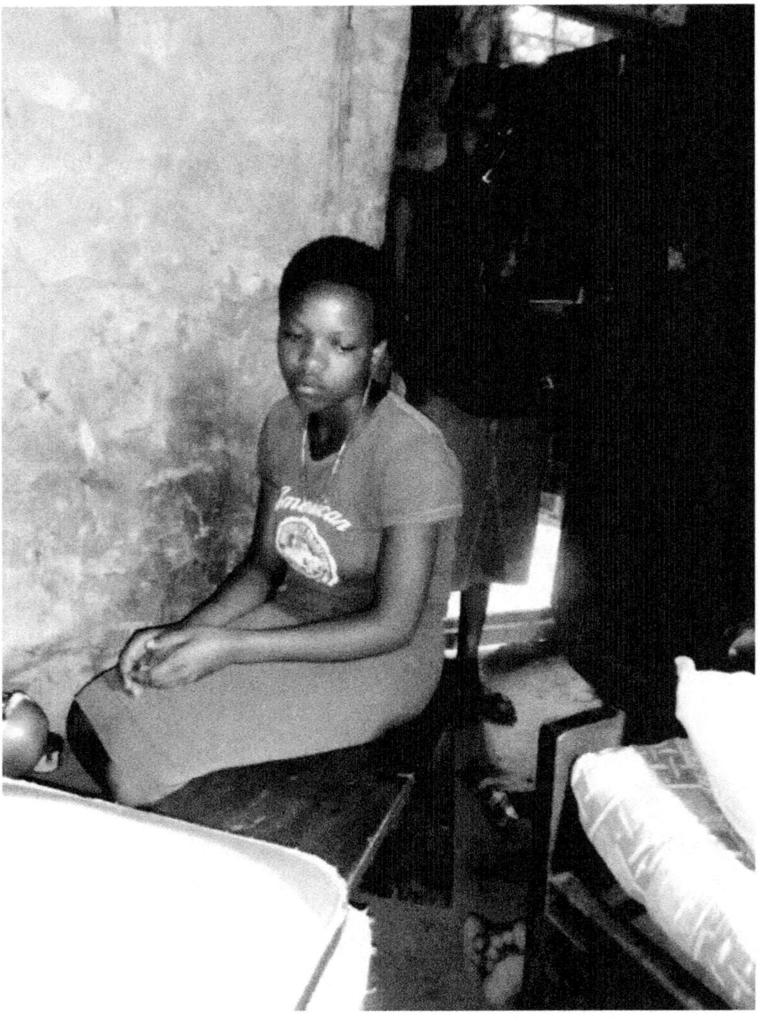

Photo 1: Mum

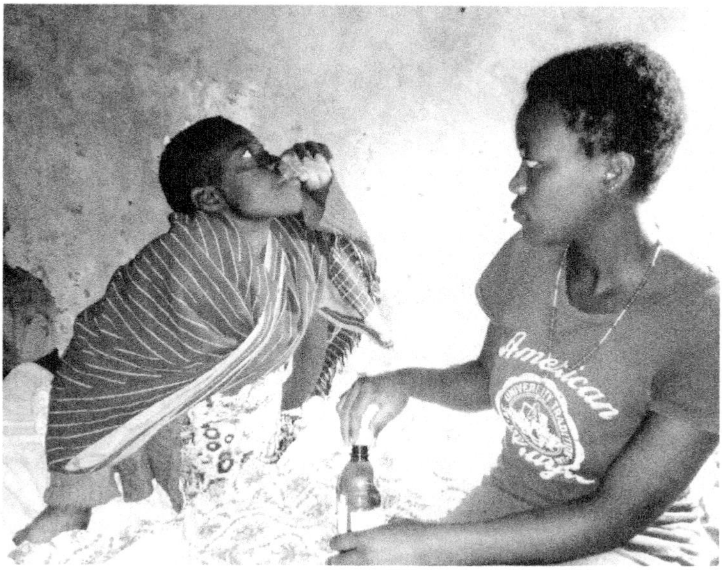

Photo 2: ***Mum and daughter***

Fortunately, we were able to give Mary morphine to keep her physical pain in check.

After Mary died, the poor children who'd been with their mother through her difficult illness and death finally got some good news. After her death a good Samaritan came and agreed to support all the children in Hospice's Give a Chance programme that fund boarding school for the children of Hospice patients who have died. They are now in school except one girl who refused; her siblings said that she got married.

5

Offering Choice and Comfort at the End of Life

Francisca Nagujja

I find it truly a challenge when I suspect that a patient has no more than a week left to live. Every time I know that I am to visit a patient like this I must ask for God's courage, patience and calmness.

Mzeei fell into this category. A 90-year-old man, he had lived with diabetes type 2 and hypertension for over 20 years. However, in the past two years he started complaining of painful limbs, describing it as multiple body aches affecting his mobility. Pain was never controlled on medications till the attending doctor requested a lumbar spine myelogram that indicated infiltrative lesion. A bone marrow biopsy was done showing multiple myeloma. He was started on chemotherapy first dose and referred to Hospice for pain control. The first visit was reviewed as a consultation by a family member who requested a home visit as they couldn't bring in the patient following severe pain and sleepless nights. He was given some morphine as per referral form and prescription. The home visit was planned for two days later.

Mzeei was a Hajji with three wives and over 23 children. He had a home care nurse attending to him when he wasn't in hospital. He looked calm in bed and was sleeping soundly. He had an NG tube (for feeding) in situ and was lying on a hospital bed.

On my reaching the home most of the family members were waiting and had so many questions to ask. Calmly, I attended to all their questions and reassured them of the Hospice role in patient care.

The family worried that morphine was making their beloved elder inactive and unconscious. They asked why the team prescribed morphine without the patient, inquired about the management plan, and wanted to know how to treat the bed sores he had developed. These were asked immediately even before getting the history of the patient. I understood how anxious and worried the family was about old Mzeei's condition.

On assessing Mzeei, he was conscious and alert on what was happening though he had slurred speech, was very weak, and had tenderness in the whole body with a bedsore in the sacral region (in between the buttocks). It was apparent to me that this man was a dying patient. The attending home care nurse gave me his observation that the patient was no longer groaning and frowning once pain medications had been started.

Following the observation, morphine was continued, with the addition of paracetamol, hibicet, metrogyl cream, and syrup lactulose. I had to do end-of-life counselling which led to an immediate debate among family members. As for whether chemotherapy should be stopped, the family was divided into those agreeing to stop and those wishing to continue. Everyone wanted to leave the NG tube inserted so this wasn't removed. I advised the family to further discuss the matter with Mzeei's long-time attending physician, since they trusted him more than me, as I had just walked in that day and was raising these vital issues. Despite the debate, the family was grateful that I'd brought up the difficult topic of end-of-life decisions. They couldn't do it by themselves, fearing the reactions from many of Mzeei's children.

Unfortunately, Mzeei died seven days later, before our next review. The family didn't take him back for chemotherapy, but the NG tube remained and they continued with pain medications which had given Mzeei such relief in his last days.

Mzee: *Mzee is a Swahili word for old man or woman.*

Hajji: *Hajji is an Arabic name for someone who has been to Mecca.*

6

Hospice Gave Hope

Martha Rabwoni

'Janine' was enrolled in Hospice nine months ago with a working diagnosis of hepatocellular carcinoma (cancer of the liver). She is 64 years old and a widow with 11 children; she now has six children: two boys and four girls; she has lost three boys and two girls.

Janine came in when her doctors gave her the diagnosis of cancer and she understood that it was not going to get any better. Her main distress was pain in the abdomen, abdominal distension and fullness.

She was given medicine and her symptoms were relieved, but she continues to fear eating because of the abdominal fullness. Janine has grown to be very emaciated and frail, but she is such a jolly lady and very appreciative for small things which are done for her.

She is a joy to visit at home; she asks for only a bun, sugar, and milk and when they are taken to her, she is so happy that she can eat the bread for a whole day. Janine does not eat much but she enjoys eating slowly and when she finishes it, the family has a reason to celebrate! She has a very caring daughter, who is a major support to her.

Janine has accepted her condition with grace; she lives one day at a time and thanks God for that day. She is very spiritual; she believes that everything is God's way to move forward. She still has her mother who is very old. She visits Janine occasionally and they give each other encouragement.

When the Hospice team visits, we find Janine sitting outside enjoying the sunshine. She appreciates interacting with the outside world and loves Hospice because they bring her visitors. When she is alone, she gets pleasure out of watching her rabbits and baby goats which she says are very beautiful animals and bring her peace.

Janine's life is nearing its end, but the time she has left is much enriched by our visits. She looks forward to the team coming, and the whole family is happy and contented with the pain control and counselling we offer to them and their dear mother.

This is palliative care at its best.

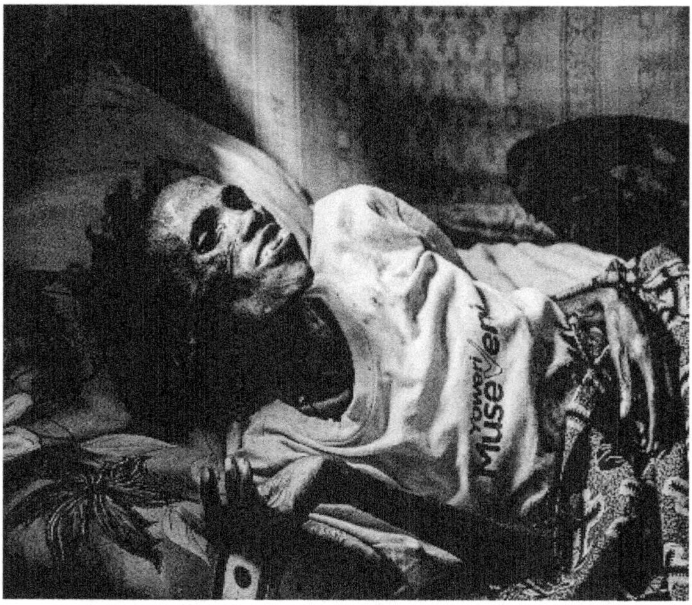

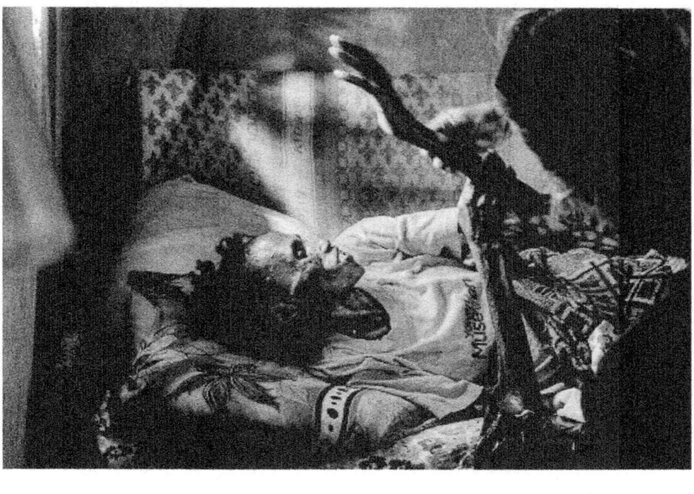

Photos 3 and 4: Janine

7

The Long Journey Home

Martha Rabwoni

'Sarah' was a 38-year-old woman with 11 children. She was a refugee from Rwanda married to a Ugandan man. She was fine and going about her work when she noticed two lumps in her left breast two years ago; she did not mind as long as they were not painful. She got pregnant again as the lumps continued to grow. Someone in the village told her that she was bewitched, and she started taking herbs, but this was no help. Eventually the lumps became so large and painful that she was unable to do her usual work as a mother.

Sarah finally decided to come to the hospital. Though Mbarara was many hours from home (367 km!), she chose the hospital there because some of her relatives were in the refugee camp in nearby Nakivale. She was brought to Mbarara Hospital where she, her three-year-old daughter and eight-month-old baby were in the care of her mother-in-law who has only one eye.

By this time Sarah was bedridden. At first, she was able to walk on one leg but the second one also got broken while she was in the hospital. Investigations showed pathological fracture of both femurs due to the previously undiagnosed cancer that had now spread throughout her body.

The patient and her mother in-law were without any resources and were living on handouts from fellow patients. Sarah was in so much pain that every movement was excruciating due to the fractures; the doctors did not know what to do to help her.

On her third day at the hospital, a nurse from Hospice came to the ward and saw Sarah. She gave her liquid morphine for the pain and some food and that night there was calm, and the poor lady finally had a night's rest. The next day the nurse returned. Sarah said her dying wish was to go back home to see her children. It was a real nightmare because she could not sit up and getting to her faraway home would be a long and difficult journey, requiring two long car rides and a boda, boda.[3] Plus, there was the issue of transport money – she had none.

Fellow patients were sympathetic and were trying to put some coins into the basket but the journey was really long and costly and they did not know whether it was a normal matatu they were collecting for or a special hire. Then the Hospice team consulted the Chief Executive of HAU, a physician himself. He understood the problem very quickly and authorized the transport to take the patient home using the Hospice van, which meant she could lie down and not have to transfer vehicles.

The patient and carer were informed of the good news. The little girl was very happy; she was looking forward to going back home to be with her father and her siblings.

On Friday evening the patient, carer, and children were brought to Hospice so that they could be ready to start the journey at 5am in the morning because of the distance. The guard at Hospice was given some money to provide the visitors with a

[3] Bicycles and motorcycle taxis.

very good meal and he made sure they had a cup of tea in the morning.

At 4:30am the driver and I, the accompanying nurse, were ready for the journey. We carefully carried the patient into the car, but every movement was punctuated by pain. I gave her a loading dose of morphine for the long journey. By 5:30 we were on our way.

The journey was horrible for the 30 minutes to drive from Hospice to Rwebikoona because of the potholes. The stretch from Rwebikoona to Ibanda was fine though the journey, which is normally; an hour, took twice as long. The young girl and her grandmother both got travel sickness because they were not used to travelling. At a certain point I was very scared that the old lady and the young girl were going to be sicker than the patient because they were having intractable vomiting. The patient and baby were fine.

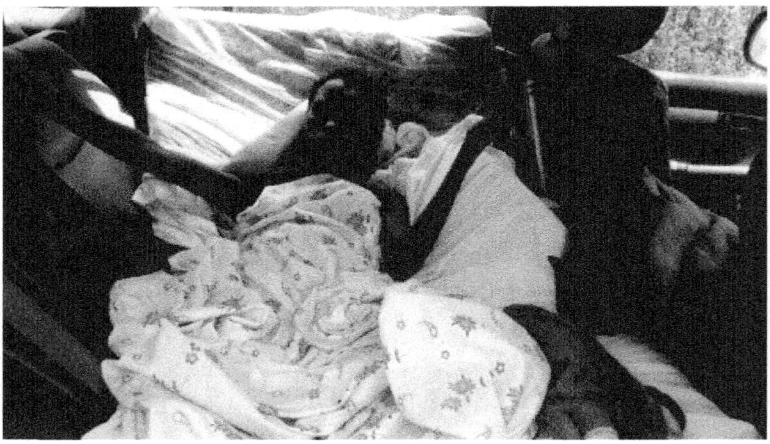

Photo 5: Sarah and her baby in the car

The worst part was from Ibanda to Kamwenge road, about 35 km. There were many potholes and the patient was in terrible pain. We had to stop so I could give her a break-through dose of morphine, which calmed the pain. Finally, at 10am we reached Fort Portal and started on the Kampala–Mubende road. This was hell on earth because it was under construction, and full of humps and bumps. We had to stop again so I could give another dose of morphine. The child and the mother-in-law also continued vomiting. It was a miserable part of the journey. Finally, we reached a stretch of good road, which was a great relief to every one of us.

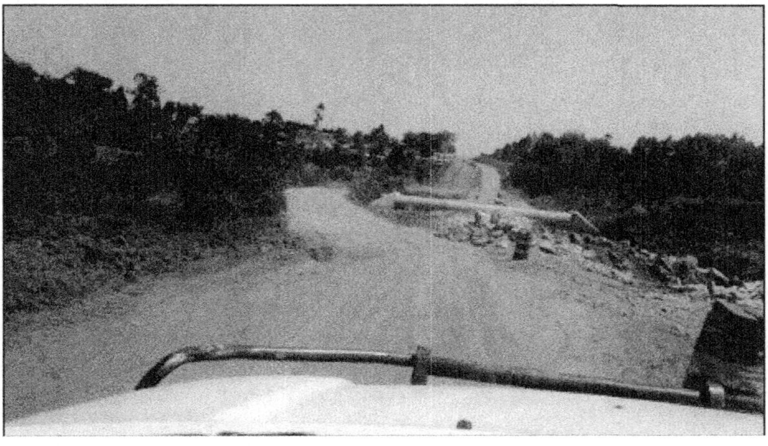

Photo 6: A stretch of good road at last!

When at last we reached Mubende town after four hours of travel, the patient and carer could not recognize their road home, so we enquired from people at the petrol station who showed us the road to Kakumiro. The road was really bad, dusty and bumpy with a lot of humps and potholes. The patient was once again in a lot of pain, so I gave her another break-through dose of morphine. We continued to enquire from passers-by for the road to Kakumiro to make sure we were still on the right track.

At last, we came to Kakumiro town. The young girl broke into a smile, and Sarah and her mother-in-law were able to direct us to the Narweyo–Kyebeya road.

It was a great relief when we finally reached home after almost 12 hours on the road; all the children were very happy to see the car which had brought their mummy.

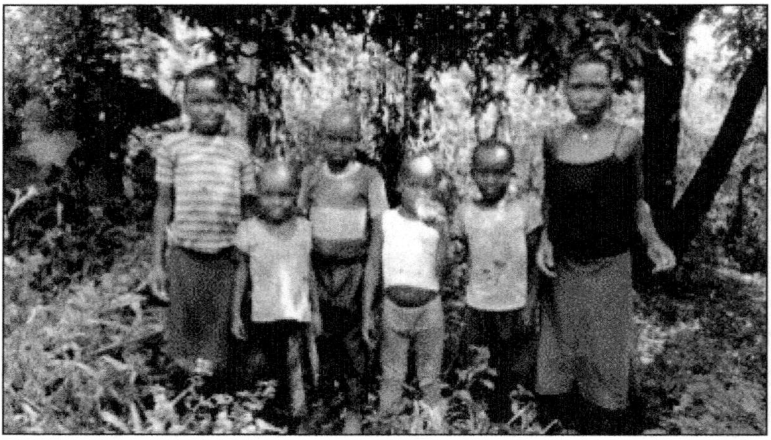

Photo 7: Sarah's children

The happiness was short-lived because mummy did not come out of the car as they had anticipated but was carried on a mattress, looking very frail and weak.

Sarah was very grateful to the entire team of Hospice for their care, love and concern for her life. She said that she was not expecting to see her children again. The old mother-in-law was also full of praises for the Hospice team having brought them back to their home.

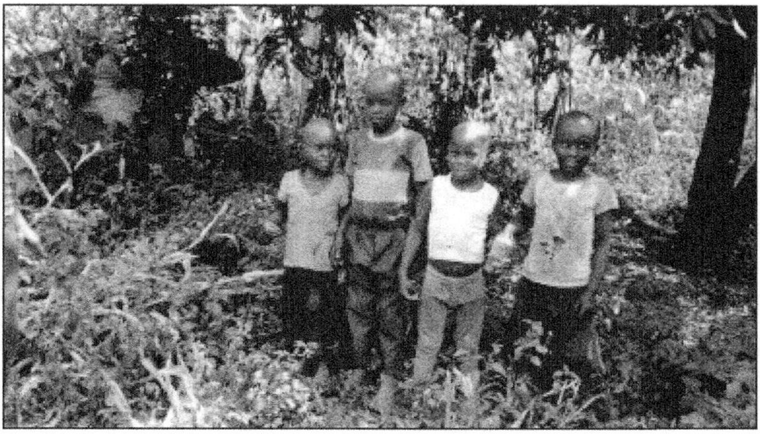

Photo 8: Four of Sarah's children, so close in age

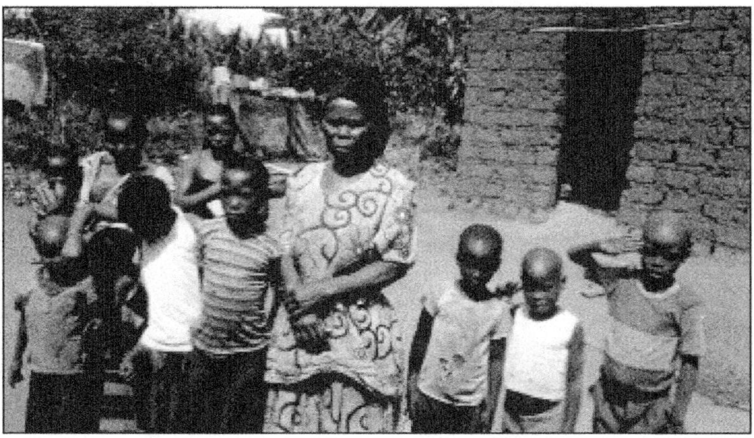

Photo 9: Mother-in-law with the children

We settled them well in their home and I gave them a supply of liquid morphine and all the instructions on how to care for Sarah. I directed them to go to Little Hospice Hoima when they need more medication. We then started our journey back home, reaching Mbarara at 10 pm in the night.

It was a long journey home, but it was worth every trouble we went through to make it.

This experience is a reminder to all of us that we can have a lasting impact on our patients and their families. We sometimes need to go a step beyond our normal duties, but if we pull together, we can do extraordinary things. This act of reuniting a dying mother with her family is still praised by not only the family but the whole community.

8

Job's Story

From One Patient to the Entire Family

Martha Rabwoni

We met a young mother at Mbarara Regional Referral Hospital with a child who was very sick and in severe pain with Stevens-Johnson syndrome, a rare and serious disorder affecting the skin and mucous membranes.

'Job' was eight years old. In his family of six children, he was the fourth born. The children were aged 3–15 years old; one had died and only the three youngest were living at home with their mother. The father was living with a new wife a bit far from their home and he was a drunkard. No one was going to school and even though they were Ugandans they were living in a refugee camp! This was so they could get some help like transport to Mbarara and live near a health centre where they could receive free treatment.

Due to a lot of pain, the staff of the hospital's children's ward referred Job to Hospice, hoping for pain control. Job's mother told us that he started with generalized abdominal swelling and pain. The child would have diarrhoea and constipation at the same time. She treated him with herbs with not much help, then someone told her that the child was being bewitched by the co-wife. As she was planning to look for the witch and had no money, the child developed vomiting and fever. He was taken to the health centre because the treatment was free.

Young Job was diagnosed with HIV and was started on Septrin (trimethoprim). He then developed blisters all over the body and became very sick. He was referred to Mbarara Regional Referral Hospital for further management, that is where we met him and his mother.

The Hospice team gave Job morphine for the pain and started him on steroids, which improved his condition. We made sure Job was given some nutrition and taught his mother how to give him food, especially during this critical moment when his mouth was very sore.

The mother was counselled about HIV status; she herself knew she was positive but not taking drugs because her husband refused to be checked. She had tested when she went to antenatal clinic for her child of three years, who was given some medicine when she was born.

We arranged with the mother to visit her at home once Job was discharged so that we could meet the father and talk to all the family about HIV and the need to test all the children. It was clear the family had multiple problems that affected their well-being: poverty, lack of knowledge on HIV and AIDS, belief in witchcraft, long distance to health Centre and an uncooperative husband/father.

On the day we visited the family we found the mother had invited the husband and his new wife and she told us that it was okay to discuss with all of them around. We brought them some more nutrition, which they needed and appreciated.

The mother had already explained to the husband about the child's sickness, and it was easy for us to start with some questions to fully understand the gaps in their knowledge; we started there to give information. We then allowed them to ask as many questions as they liked. One of the father's questions was: 'will Job grow up to be a man and have children' since he had some sores on his penis? We explained that it was possible as long as he takes his drugs and continues to get better as he had already improved quite a bit.

The father agreed to go for a check-up regarding HIV status with the new wife and the mother agreed to take the other children for testing.

Job continued to improve. We later stopped by the health clinic to which we'd referred the family. The nurses told us that the family has now been registered for ARV treatment and the mother of Job was their friend.

When we visited towards Christmas, Job had improved so much, and the other children were all looking well. Job runs almost a kilometre to go and call his mother from the garden to tell her that his friends had come. We brought them some Christmas treats which were very welcomed on that hot day in the garden.

So, in addition to addressing Job's presenting condition in the hospital, we were able to help the entire family. We helped them start on HIV treatment, dispelled the fear of witchcraft and connected them to the nearest health centre for ongoing treatment. Mother went back to work in her garden and the family had some food to eat to keep them healthy. Father being a drunkard still needed a lot of time of persuading to bring him on board, but at least he listened to what we had to say.

All this was done in love, care, patience, and persistence with the family and continued reviewing and explaining.

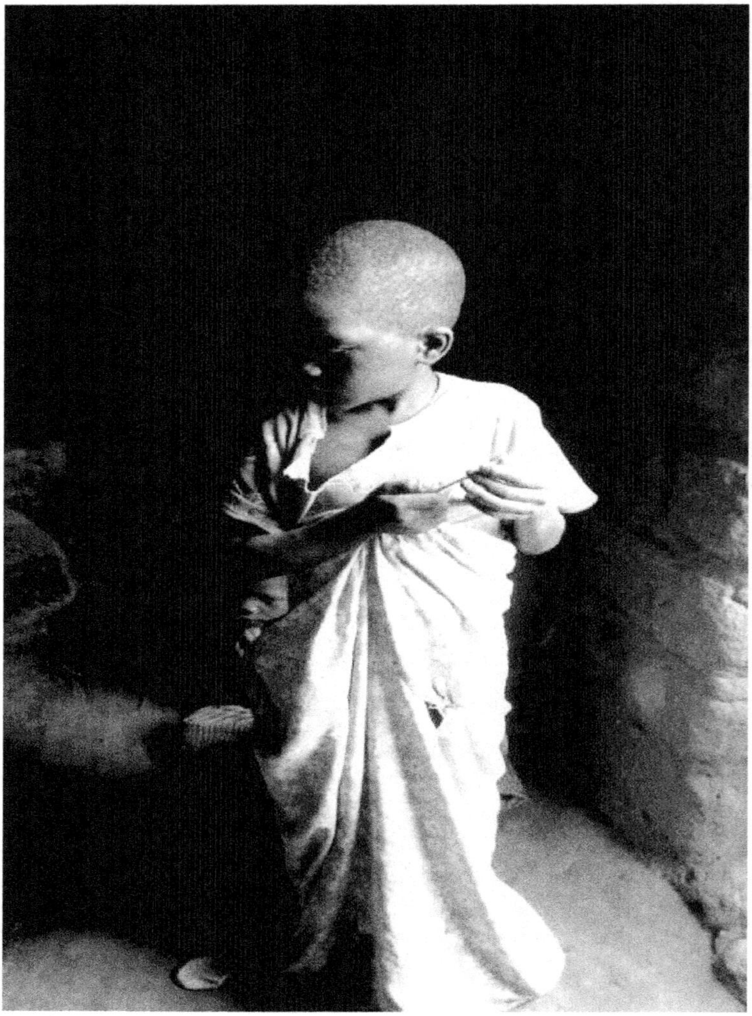

Photo 10: Job: Before treatment

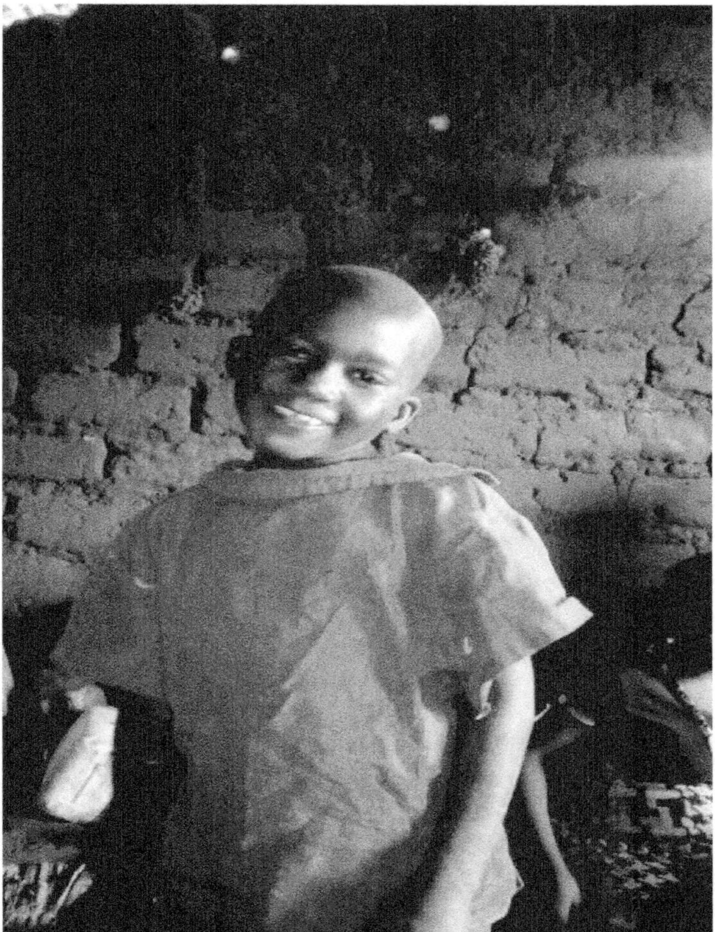

Photo 11: Job: After treatment

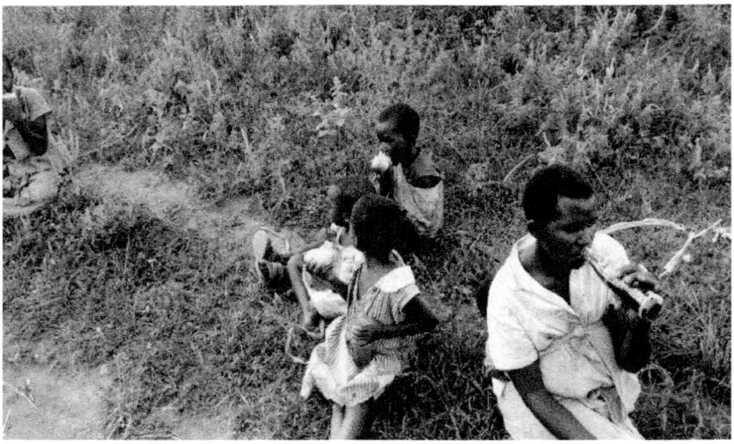

Photo 12: Family in garden

9

Caring Gave Me a Second Chance at Life

Martha Rabwoni

'Jane,' 19 years old, was admitted to the Hospice programme with HIV, pulmonary tuberculosis, and breathlessness. She had a history of not taking her drugs regularly. She looked very unwell, with nausea and vomiting, chest pain, cough, loss of weight, and hunger.

Jane was married to a man whom she did not love; they were now separated. She was still annoyed because she had had an abortion during their time together as a couple; she was also thinking that the man infected her with HIV. Her mother was mentally ill, her father had died, and she was living with a brother with whom she did not get on well.

Jane was started on anti-tuberculosis treatment and was encouraged to take her ARVs for HIV regularly. She had very little money and didn't know how she would afford to come to Hospice. Once on the Hospice Program, the team allocated her money for food and transport. We visited Jane monthly to make sure she was adhering to her treatment. With time, Jane improved so much that she was weaned off the programme and transferred to the ART (HIV treatment) programme near her home area. She was able to live with her mother who was on treatment for mental illness; they were fine together at that point.

One year later Jane came back and told us that she had been working as house help and was raped some months earlier. Since then, she had not had her period. She looked unkempt, was talking incoherently, seemed very dehydrated and was carrying stones and broken glasses in a bag. Jane's feet were swollen, and she said that she had walked a long distance. On further investigations, we determined she was indeed pregnant.

The Hospice Team arranged for Jane to be taken to the psychiatric ward for assessment, where the staff welcomed her as a long-lost friend. They told us they knew her well; she was on treatment but had absconded. Jane was admitted and restarted on psychiatric treatment, which helped her immensely. She was discharged and we took her to antenatal clinic where she was followed up during pregnancy. We talked to one of her relatives to arrange a place where she could stay while attending ante natal and psychiatric clinic. She was taken to a paternal aunt who agreed to take care of her.

We continued to take care of Jane and to encourage the aunt to make sure she took her drugs regularly and ate well. When the aunt saw that Jane's pregnancy was developing she chased her away; she was afraid of what would happen if labour started in the middle of the night. They lived very far from any health centre, and we had emphasized the importance of prevention of mother to child. The Hospice team helped Jane connect with a friend near the hospital who was willing to take care of her until the baby arrived.

On 25 November 2013 Jane delivered a healthy baby girl. Everyone was happy for her, and she loved her baby. She was given baby clothes and other items. She was now very keen on taking her treatment regularly. Hospice continued to support her by giving her money for food and transport to collect her drugs.

As Jane continued with treatment and ongoing counselling, she developed insight into her sickness. She came and told us that she as much as she loves her child, she was unable to care for her. We could see that the baby was not putting on weight, despite being HIV negative. The baby was hungry all the time. So, we found someone willing to take on Jane's baby. Jane agreed, so long as she would bring the baby to Hospice to visit the mother on a monthly basis.

Jane decided to go back to her mother's place to live and continue with subsistence farming and to care for her mother. She came to Hospice once a month to pick her drugs and see her baby. This way the Hospice team was able to keep track of Jane and ensure that she was maintaining her treatment and was continuing to maintain the stability she had found.

Jane was facing multiple physical problems and social problems that affected not only her but also the family and friends who were caring for her. With the help of Hospice, these issues were identified and addressed, and she is now able to live a more productive and happier life! The only problem is that Jane's baby has no paternal relatives which is a situation that still has to be addressed.

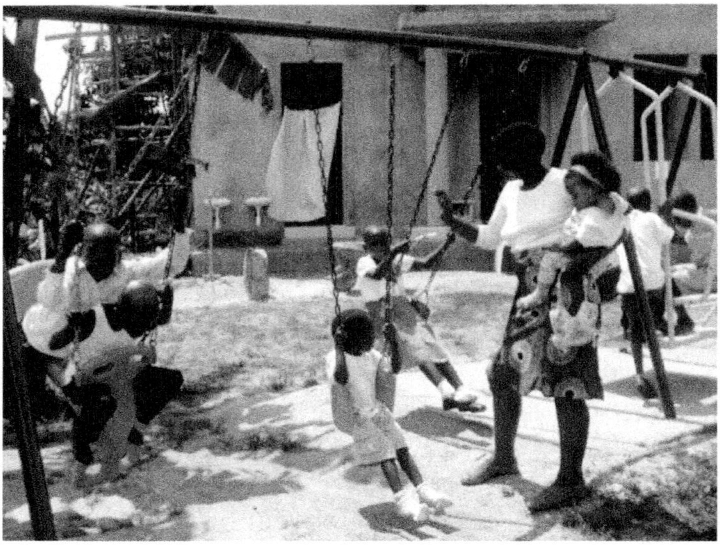

Photo 13: Jane carrying her baby
and playing with other children

10

From Pain and Suffering to Stability

Martha Rabwoni

'Margery' was a fine girl of 13 years, the first born of four children: two boys and two girls. She was growing well, studying well, but due to poverty in the family she was still in Primary Four.

In 2015, Margery started complaining of headache and pain in the eyes with blurred vision. She was taken to a clinic and got treatment for her eyes. Two months later she developed pain in her legs and backache with numbness in the toes. These symptoms soon disappeared; she was well and went back to school.

In June 2016, Margery's symptoms came back and the pain was so much that she was unable to sit. She could only lie down and cry day and night from the pain and even developed seizures. She developed lower limb paralysis. The parents took the child to a church for healing prayers where they found someone who told them to go to hospital. She was taken to a nearby hospital, from which she was referred to Mbarara Regional Referral Hospital.

The people in her church collected the money to enable Margery to travel to Mbarara. The father was alcoholic and had diabetes; and the mother was solely in charge of the family. When she brought Margery to hospital, the rest of the children were taken to live with their grandmother who was very old. The neighbours came in to help the old lady.

When Hospice met Margery, her mother was trying to figure out how to get money to get her a CT-scan; she was very distressed, hungry, and angry and wanted to run away. The Hospice team clerked the child and put her on the Programme. Thank God we had funding from DFID, which paid for a CT-scan of the brain which was very expensive. The CT showed a tumour and Margery had surgery to remove it; unfortunately, after the operation she became completely unconscious.

Margery remained unconscious at the hospital for some time. She developed bed sores and her mother, very discouraged, wanted to go back home and give up on the struggle. Then one day, Margery woke up. She was talking in an uncoordinated way and was unable to see but was conscious and able to speak.

We continued to support the mother with food, pampers, and counselling. Margery was still in pain which was controlled using morphine. The doctors on the ward were feeling they were fighting a losing battle, as Margery's condition did not improve. She was discharged and sent to an organization which cares for disabled children. We transported Margery there; by then Margery had developed hydrocephalus.

The mother was taught exercises which she could help Margery do at home and the Hospice team continued supporting her with pain relief and home visits. Margery's home was hard to reach due to poor roads and hilly area. The mother would carry her on her back to take her home because the car could not reach the homestead.

Sometime after she returned home, we visited Margery. She was sitting up in bed with her siblings around her and she looked happy. Then with time Margery's condition improved somewhat. She was able to feel when she wanted to go to the toilet and her wounds from the bedsores healed.

Margery was now able to crawl and do some simple house chores like removing beans from the pod. The mother was now very happy and relaxed even though during this time her husband died due to diabetes. Margery was eventually able to talk with the mother like an adult. She was still unable to walk but the pain was gone.

Just recently Margery came to Hospice with her mother for review. She is able to walk with an aid even though she cannot see properly.

Margery was helped by the Hospice team throughout her journey through pain and serious disability to a stable life at home with her mother. We arranged for DFID funds to pay for her CT-scan, successfully managed her pain through morphine and other medications, and provided comfort and support to both mother and daughter by visiting her at home. It was good for the people in the village not to give up on a sick child because they also contributed to making Margery better by contributing to her transport to hospital.

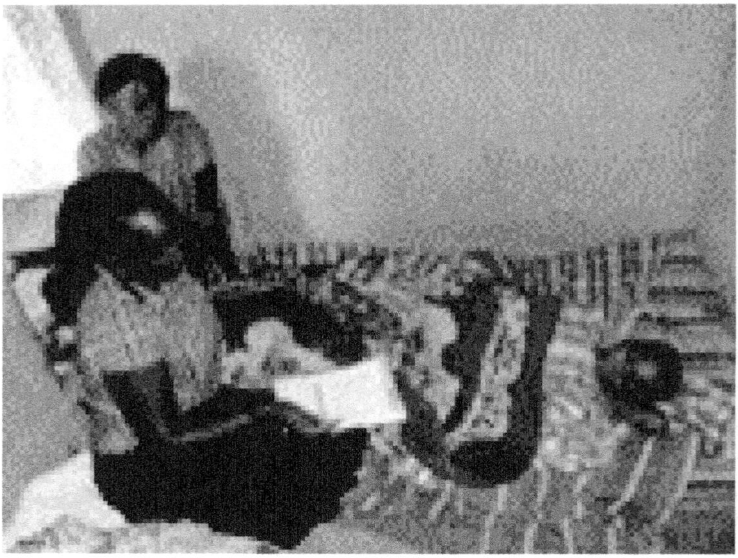

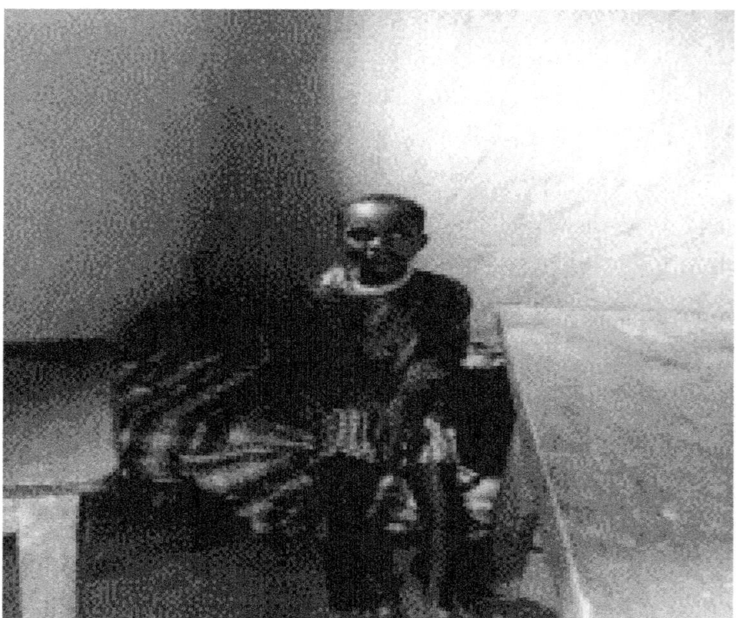

Photos 14 and 15: Margery

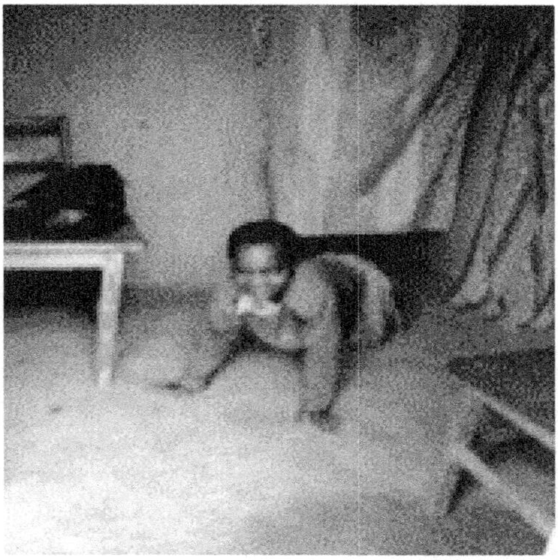

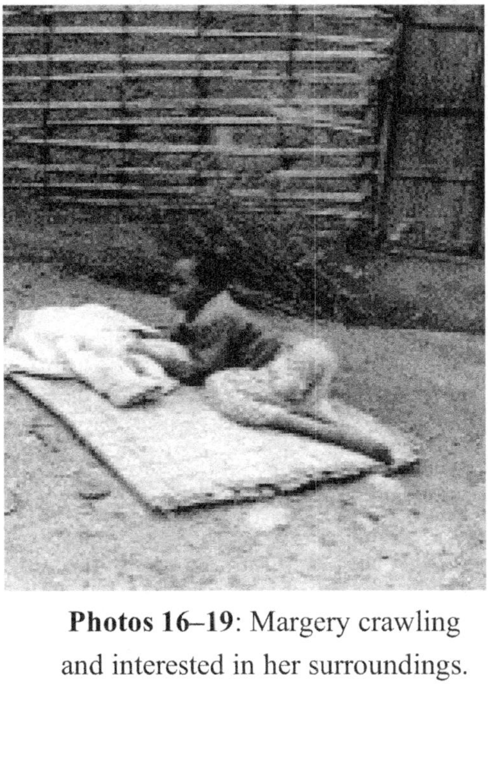

Photos 16–19: Margery crawling and interested in her surroundings.

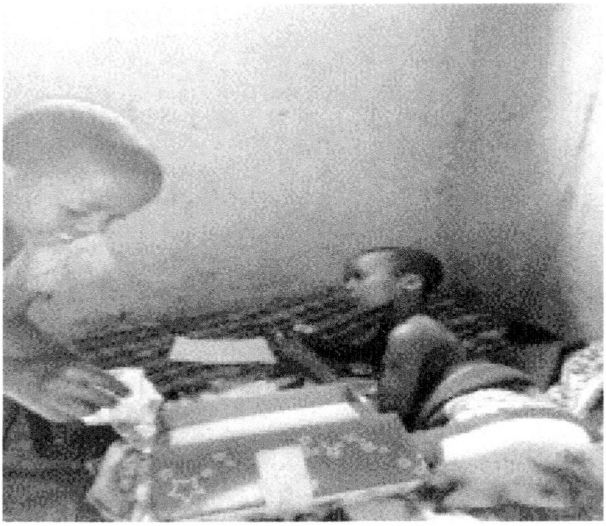

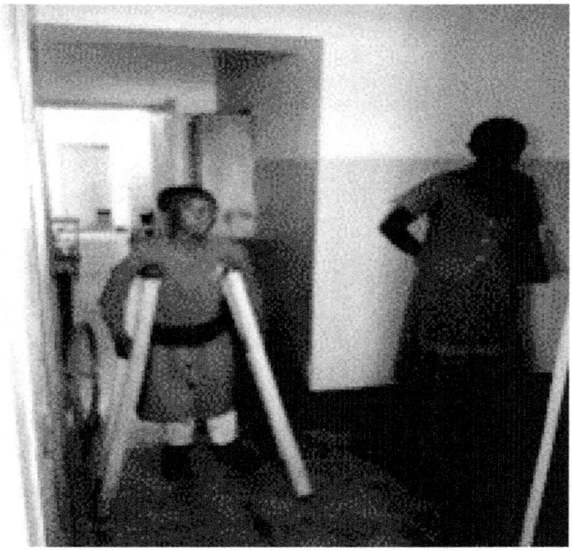

11

Who Took Away My Pain?

Martha Rabwoni

'Saturday' is a young man of 23 years. He is the second born in a family of four: two girls and two boys. The family lost their father to HIV/AIDS who left them when they were very young; their mother brought them up alone in spite of being very sick herself. She was happy; her boys had grown up and they would be her protector.

The brother became sick and died suddenly in 2013, leaving Saturday as the eldest child. Some time later, Saturday developed a painless lump on his neck, which he ignored. The swelling continued to grow and became painful. As it increased in size, the family used local herbs with no improvement.

The pain became so bad that at one time Saturday wanted to commit suicide and he was taken to Kampala International Hospital. He was treated and sent to Mbarara Regional Referral Hospital. Investigations were done, a biopsy revealed Non-Hodgkin's Lymphoma, and he was being worked up to be started on chemotherapy.

He was told to do more investigations but the family had run out of money. They had sold their plot of land so had nothing to sell. So, Saturday went back home and waited for death. The pain was too much, he was in misery and death could not come fast enough to put an end to his suffering.

As the mother was sharing her woes with a friend, she was directed to Hospice. She could not wait and used her last coins to travel to our site. She arrived at the end of the last day of the week when all staff were tired and looking forward to a restful weekend.

She narrated her story, but her home was beyond the catchment area – 64 km from Hospice. When we explained this, she broke down and cried terribly. Some consultations were done and it was agreed that she should be given some analgesics and be visited the next day, by the staff who was on duty, even though the distance was very far. The lady went back home with some hope. She directed the staff and promised to be on the roadside to take the team home when they arrived.

The next day I set off to visit Saturday with the driver, it was a rainy day and when we reached the spot where we had agreed to meet, she was not there. We forgave her because of the rain, called her on phone and she said that she was on her way. We followed the path she had told us. People on the way were very helpful in directing us towards her home. As we were approaching the path where we were supposed to branch off, the dusty road was graded the day before and it was like a garden to plant beans!

My heart missed a beat because I knew what was coming. The driver was very quiet. We drove in silence and the skidding started and immediately I told the driver to stop and let me out with my bag so that I could walk to the patients' home. Meanwhile, he had to find people to help him get the car out of the mud.

The walk was a long one with hills to climb and finally I found the home with the help of the neighbours. I found Saturday lying on the floor with his whole head and neck swollen. I was shocked and did not know what to do, as his condition was so serious. His breathing was difficult and he was groaning in pain. I greeted the mother and the sister who looked very exhausted.

I gave Saturday a dose of morphine and an injection of steroids. I clerked him and by the time I finished, Saturday asked the mother, Mum are you preparing a cup of tea for the visitor? It brought a smile to the mother's face because this was the first time Saturday was able to think of another person besides his pain and himself. Saturday's main distress was to die without a child and before he finished building his house.

By the time I finished the sun had come out and Saturday's pain had subsided. I gave them the drugs for pain and told them that we will come and see them in four days' time because we have an outreach on that route. I also advised them to return for chemotherapy at Mbarara Regional Referral Hospital. I said Hospice will pay for investigations and transport.

When we visited Saturday on our way to the outreach, he was at church with his bottle of morphine and all his drugs. He knew he was improving because he had walked by himself to go to church. He was reviewed by the doctor and was planning to follow my earlier instructions of going to Mbarara for chemotherapy.

One week later the mother came to the office and told us that Saturday was dying. He was unable to breath. The team rushed again to Saturday's home and brought him to hospital. A tracheostomy was done and investigations were done and he was started on chemotherapy. We continued visiting him and supporting the mother with food and drinks for the patient.

Saturday was now worried about the hole in his throat (tracheostomy) but with time it was removed and Saturday was given a mirror to look at himself. He could not believe himself because the person who looked back at him was completely different and that is how he was feeling – the tumour had drastically reduced, the pain was gone. On discharge Saturday came himself to say thank you to the team at Hospice who saved his life. He is still receiving the treatment but he has hope and he has a life to live. The mother's tears were dried.

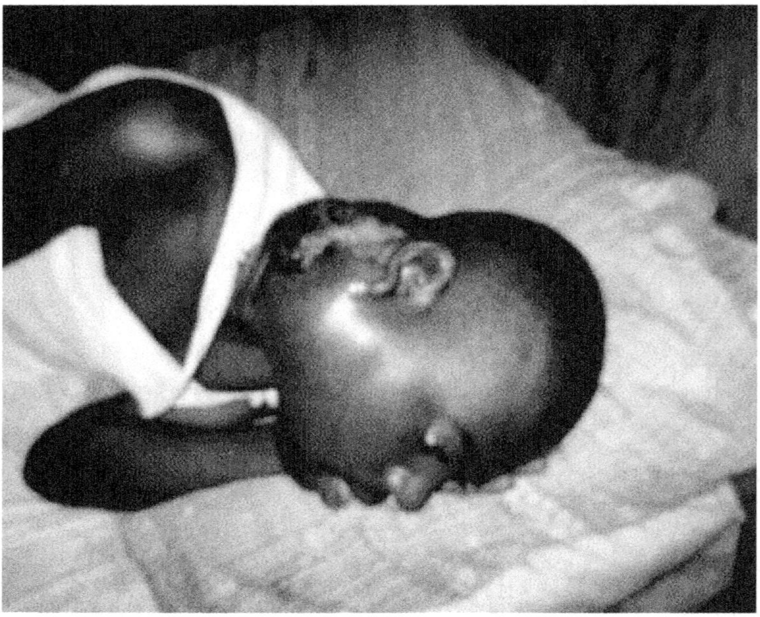

Photo 20: Saturday: before intervention

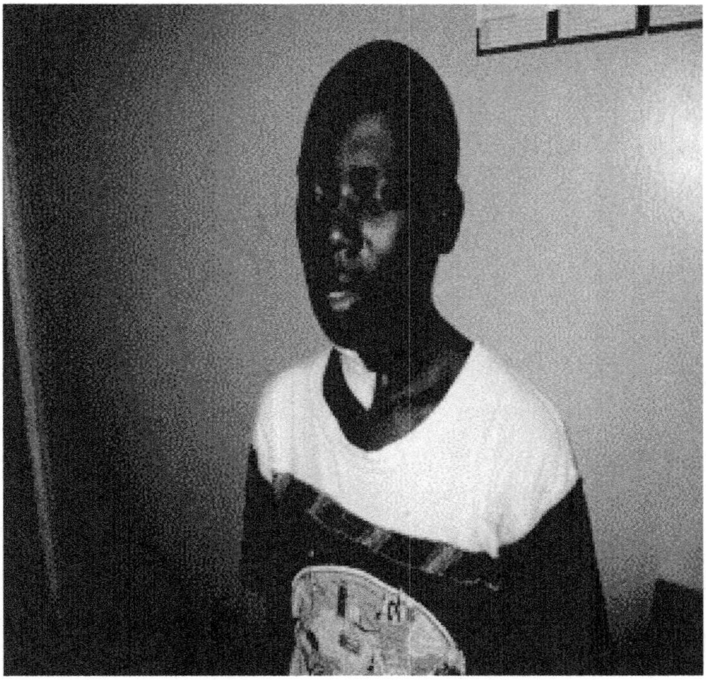

Photo 21: Saturday: after intervention.

12

A Young Girl's Road to Healing

Martha Rabwoni

'Maureen' is a five-year-old girl, the first born of three children. She was born on 7 July 2010. Maureen has been sick for a long time. She was born with an umbilical hernia which was repaired.

At the time she had a swelling on one thigh and a biopsy was done which revealed Rhabdo-myosarcoma (cancer of the left thigh). She was started on chemotherapy. Maureen was referred to the Hospice staff when she was on the third cycle of chemotherapy. She was miserable with pain, had infection, her temperature was high and she was not talking. The poor child looked very sick and despondent.

The mother was distressed because the child was not well, she was early into her next pregnancy and they had no money to buy food in the hospital. Plus, she had left a young child at home who had just been weaned from the breast and she did not know how the husband was coping with the home chores without her.

The only thing the mother wanted was to get money and take the child home. They were given a drink and the child was given some Paracetamol syrup to reduce the temperature and Amoxyl syrup for the infection. We encouraged the mother to give the child plenty of fluids.

They were given money for transport after intensive counselling and encouraged to come back after one week. Then the mother felt better as she went back home. She returned a week later with Maureen who was looking much better and was able to play and smile.

So far Maureen has had 18 cycles of chemotherapy. The swelling is reducing and Maureen has gone back to school.

On 21 September 2015 another baby girl was born in the family, who they named Anne. The whole family is very happy with the new arrival. When the team visited with Dr Anne, she was also very happy because this was the first time seeing a baby named Anne since she came to Uganda. She was given a nice small sweater.

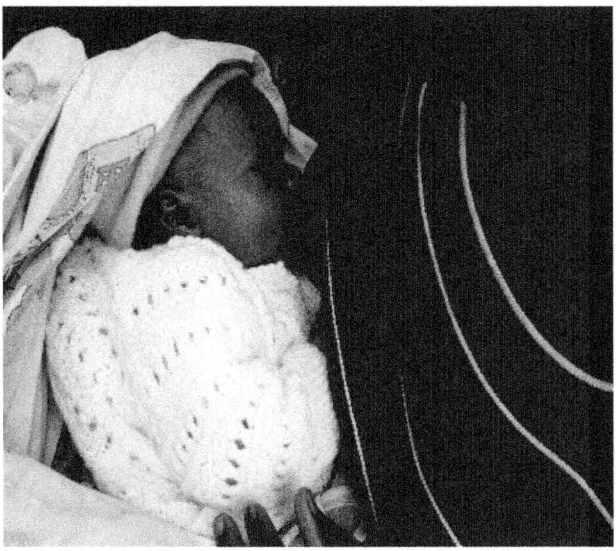

Photo 22: Anne in her sweater

13

A Palliative Care Success Story

Martha Rabwoni

'Angel,' a beautiful 14-year-old, was referred by Mbarara Regional Referral Hospital to Hospice in early April 2016 with a working diagnosis of osteoarthritis after fracturing her leg while playing netball at school, where she was in Primary Seven.

Angel's health history showed she'd had pains in the legs which were treated and she'd been discharged back home when this tragedy happened. On enrolment in Hospice, she was experiencing multiple pains that got the attention of everyone in the hospital. Angel spent all day undressed because any touch on her skin caused a lot of pain.

Being young, she was afraid of any intervention, but her wish was to control her pain. Angel also had a swelling on the hip joint that stopped her from sitting. Her physical pains were managed with morphine, but the delay in healing and continual swelling, especially given her youth, were a concern for which she needed ongoing counselling.

A multidisciplinary team investigated the swelling for possible rhabdomyosarcoma, lymphoma, or osteosarcoma. The diagnosis was finally Rhabdomyosacroma, a rare cancer of the soft tissue. Angel was started on chemotherapy and showed some improvement over a month. She was even discharged back home in the process of awaiting her next dose of chemotherapy. The Hospice team visited her at home and found her smiling.

Angel is the second born of six children of which the eldest is 16 and youngest three years. Her mother was pregnant and was the main carer. It was difficult for her to lift Angel on her own and she had many other duties as mother of six. We supported her in getting a helper with whom she could make shifts in caring for Angel. It took us some time to help the mother understand her child's diagnosis since all she wanted was for her sweet Angel get cured. She even reached time when she could not provide the painkillers to her child and resorted to prayers while alone.

As a team we never gave up till when she understood and appreciated the severe illness of her daughter and the importance of easing her pain through medication.

Angel's wish was to stay in hospital until she got better. On returning there to receive her second dose of chemotherapy, her condition worsened. She developed multiple swellings, with generalized oedema, and severe pain which was managed well. However, at this time we realized that chemotherapy was not of any use; we advocated for it to be stopped which was done. We counselled the mother who requested her daughter not be discharged since she was scared of any eventualities at home, which was far from health facilities. This was respected by oncology team, and Angel remained hospitalized. The Hospice team followed up with her at the hospital and supported the mother and family.

In addition to physical pain, Angel had a lot of emotional pain which the team addressed through talk therapy. When she realized that her drugs were stopped, Angel requested an explanation. However hurtful it was, this gave the team the opportunity to explain that her condition was incurable, after a long period of her not wanting to hear this but focusing only on curing her disease. In simple language we explained to her that she needed to prepare for the end of her life. Friends and teachers visited her for final farewells.

During her last days when asked what she wanted, Angel asked to be told stories about Hospice and its founder and wanted perfume and even a doll. Even though very weak and bedridden, she somehow found the energy to play with her three-year-old brother. She was a very special patient, engaging with other patients and encouraging them to continue their treatment since she knew she didn't have the chance to live longer.

Angel died peacefully in late July. The family was also at peace since we gave them the chance to appreciate their child, smile with her even when she was sick, and prepare for her death. The team was comfortable and even the oncology team felt counselled and prepared for this special beautiful Angel to leave them.

May Your Soul Rest in peace. You're still in our hearts and we will miss you.

14

'In the Next Three Days, the Maggots Were No More'

A Story of Hospice and Palliative Care

Natuhwera Germans

'Nellie' is an 89-year-old widow. She was brought to Little Hospice Hoima (LHH) in November 2020 by her children. She had no medical document as she had never before sought medical care for her condition. She had a fungating tumour in the left armpit for over three years. A fungating wound is a wound in the skin marked by ulcerations (breaks on the skin surface) and necrosis (death of living tissue) and often has a bad smell. Of surprise to note is that she had never disclosed this to any of her family members. Her daughter who was visiting saw blood stains on her bed and asked her mum what was going on. Only then, did she learn that her mother had a tumour.

When asked why she kept the wound a secret, she answered, 'I never wanted to disturb my children... I have secretly been massaging it with warm water hoping it would heal but it has refused...' Her daughter added 'She always kept herself covered in clothes, she showered privately and always ensured no one saw her. We can't imagine this … it's really very scary.'

The patient in fact threatened to curse this daughter if she dared disclose her condition to the other children. Terrified by the state and size of the tumour, the daughter informed the brothers and sisters. The son fortunately learned about LHH and brought her there that November.

In a discussion with a Hospice clinician about her needs, Nellie affirmed several times that she was not comfortable with any futile intervention, including operation, though her children very much wanted to know the nature or cause of the tumour and were ready to finance her care. The clinician provided information on the condition and possible interventions to the family. Their decision was to remain on palliative care only at LHH.

The clinicians cleaned Nellie's wound and took out several maggots; they couldn't get all of them out. They also treated Nellie's pain and taught the daughter how to take care of the tumour at home. After three days, the daughter called and informed the Hospice team that the maggots were no more and the foul-smelling discharge had reduced.

Two weeks later, the Hospice team visited the patient at home. As Christmas was fast approaching, the team brought a Merry Christmas food pack from HAU. At that home visit, they reviewed and changed Nellie's pain medicines, as Nellie was still in pain. The food pack gave her joy, but she most needed pain relief. She was started on oral liquid morphine (available to Ugandans free of charge, made at Hospice Africa Uganda in Kampala and delivered through the National Medical Stores to local pharmacies) as well as other pain medicines.

In a situation where a patient does not want aggressive interventions, the Hospice and palliative care team intensifies education and counselling for the patient and family. The goal of care is centred on relieving the patient's symptoms and supporting patient and family through the end-of life-period.

'Nellie' was able to enjoy her final Christmas in comfort at home, pain-free and surrounded by her family. The LHH team visited several times more, to monitor Nellie's symptoms and help mother and family prepare for her passing. Nellie died peacefully three weeks after Christmas. The family remains ever grateful for the loving care she received from the Hospice team.'

15

Kay's Experience

Living with Breast Cancer

Natuhwera Germans and Elizabeth Namugambe

'Kay' is a 32-year-old total orphan born in a family of three siblings. She was referred to Little Hospice Hoima (LHH) in July 2014 with suspected cancer of the right breast following a complaint of a small lump in the right breast.

Kay had earlier noticed a painless lump which she ignored and never sought medical attention. Later, the lump increased in size and prompted her to visit a private clinic. A breast scan was run, and treatment was given with no improvement. In July 2014, she decided to go to Hoima Regional Referral Hospital. She was given treatment, but it did not help. In August, she started on herbal medicines; they did not help either.

Kay then shared her condition with a friend who fortunately was a daughter to a Community Volunteer Worker (CVW) attached to LHH. Upon being alerted by her daughter, the CVW immediately referred Kay to LHH. On her initial visit to LHH, Kay reported insect bite-like pains, a lump and bloody discharge from the right nipple. She surely needed a biopsy to rule out cancer of the breast.

Kay was living with the father of her one year and eight-months-old baby; the father was a truck driver. Kay had studied up to ordinary secondary level 4 and was working as a guest house attendant. She and the baby's father would not be able to afford the biopsy, transport costs, costs of investigations, and treatment at Uganda Cancer Institute (UCI). While Kay was at home mobilizing funds for the biopsy, neighbours unfortunately convinced her that her disease would progress faster if she accepted a biopsy. She was instead encouraged to continue herbal medicines on which she reported some improvement in spite of the persistent pain and the lump.

The palliative care team at LHH did not relent because they had seen many patients with nasty outcomes having followed the path Kay was on. They intensified their follow-up and counselling until Kay accepted the biopsy, three months later. In May 2015, using funds from the patient support fund at LHH, Kay was supported to go to UCI. A series of investigations, including biopsy, were done and adenocarcinoma (cancer) of the breast was confirmed. In June 2015, she was referred from UCI to Hoima Regional Referral Hospital for a mastectomy and the following month, July 2015, she started on chemotherapy at UCI.

LHH continued to provide Kay with financial and psychosocial support. She experienced a lot of distress during this season of medical interventions. She had post-operation pain, swelling of the right arm, and hair loss due to the chemotherapy, abdominal fullness and the feeling of disfigurement, having lost one breast. She was one of the lucky ones that got a prosthetic breast.

While all this was going on in her body, Kay was also suffering emotionally and psychologically. She missed her son during the hospital admissions. Her sister would not take care of him so he had to be with the father, yet Kay wasn't trusting enough that the boy's father could look after the baby. When she started chemotherapy, she felt she could not afford the treatment as well as take care of her son, which greatly worried her. To make matters worse, her son's father later deserted them and she lost her job.

Kay underwent treatment at UCI, improved, and was later discharged home on oral tamoxifen, which she still takes daily. Her main concern now is itching at the mastectomy scar. She continues to receive palliative care at LHH for pain and symptom control, and Hospice still supports her with transport to attend her reviews at UCI every after three months. Fortunately, she is in a new relationship, living with her baby and is happy.

16

Going the Extra Mile for a Palliative Care Patient

Dorcus Aciiro

'Jackie' was a 42-year-old lady, living in a Kampala suburb on the shores of Lake Victoria, who came to Hospice Africa Uganda in 2018. She had a nasal tumour which brought her unimaginable pain. At the time the palliative care team first saw her she was in misery and a prescription of oral liquid morphine was inevitable because all the pain medications she had tried had proved ineffective for her pain.

While the physical pain from the horrible nasal tumour was a prominent feature in Jackie's daily life, it is her psychosocial issues that were more troubling for her. Jackie was a widow. Her husband had passed on several years before Hospice first met her and she was fending for five young children by herself. She had managed to secure a job as a cook in a nursery school. With her monthly wage of 20 euros, she struggled very much to balance it all. It is difficult to imagine how for years Jackie managed to meet the costs of essentials like food, the school fees for her children's education, and many other expenses of daily living.

When Jackie fell sick, her world started spiralling out of control. She could no longer cook at school because the smoke in the school kitchen irritated her nasal tumour so much that she found it extremely difficult to breathe. Jackie's relatives were not supportive, and she felt a sense of hopelessness. Amid the tragedy of her difficult job whilst unwell, Jackie's teenage son developed a medical complication that required surgery, and her daughter was involved in a serious accident that left her hand deformed and rendered this extra pair of hands unable to participate in most domestic chores. This simply increased the workload Jackie had to face every day.

Jackie had saved a little money and with it, she had bought a small plot of land and started construction of what she hoped to be a humble family home. However, as the disease that plagued her progressed, she spent all her savings on chemotherapy and other expensive treatments. This inevitably brought her home-building project to an abrupt halt.

Despite her deteriorating health, Jackie continued to endure a smoke-filled school kitchen because her greatest fear was that her family would be evicted from the house if the rent dues piled up.

In the course of HAU's caregiving to Jackie, we became keenly aware that her main distress was her living condition. To address her plight, HAU's social workers wrote up Jackie's story with a special appeal for Good Samaritans to come to her rescue. A generous gift of 500 Euros, approximately 2,075,000 UGX, was given to HAU by a donor to help Jackie complete the construction of her house. With that donation through HAU, the family purchased iron sheets, timber, and other roofing materials and covered the costs of labour for roofing the house.

While it is sad to report that Jackie passed on a few days after the completion of her new house, her children are now living in it and are at peace because they know that their mother's dying wish was granted. They have the security of a safe place they call home.

Although the building of houses for poor patients is not HAU's core mandate, our holistic approach and our acknowledgment of the multiple problems our patients face, compels us to go out of our way to address the extraordinary yet ordinary needs of families.

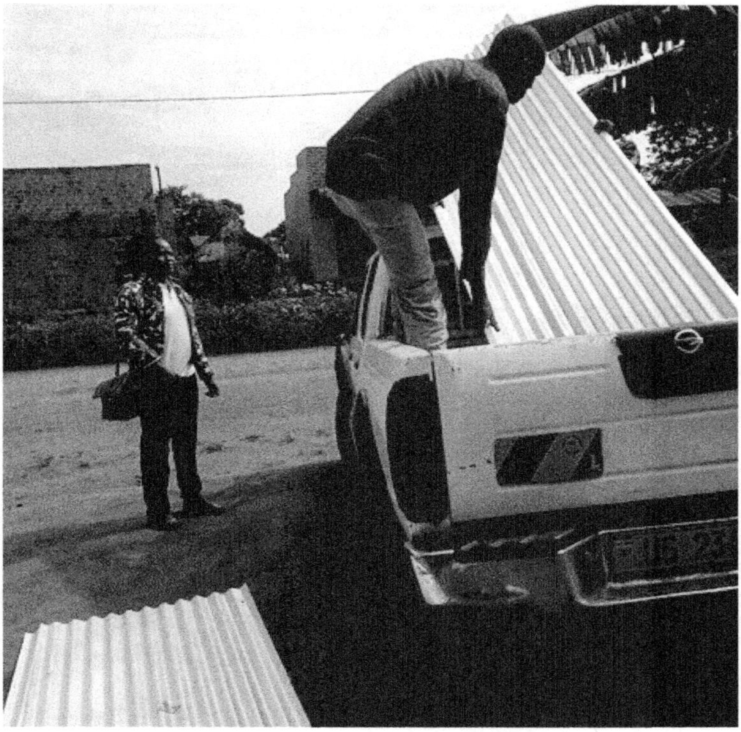

Photo 23: Iron sheets were procured, and ferried by the Hospice vehicle

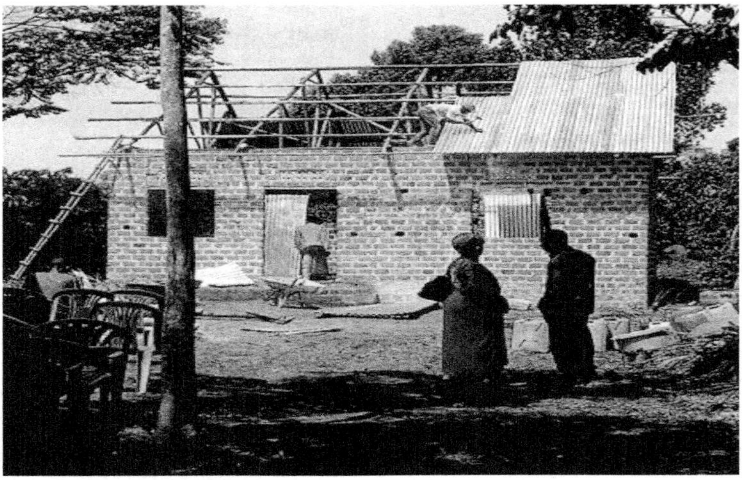

Photo 24: Jackie's incomplete house being roofed

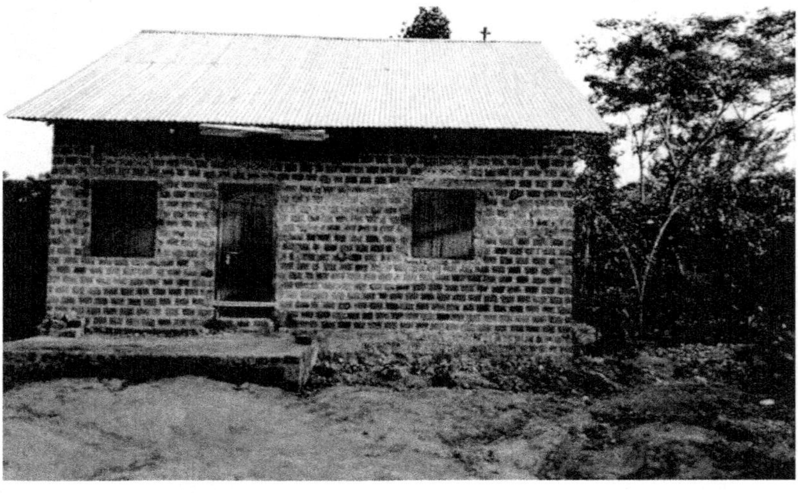

Photo 25: Jackie's house after it was completed

17

A Story of How the HAU Team Thinks Outside the Box

Kampala HAU Clinical Team

'Immaculate' is a 29-year-old woman from the Amuria district of Uganda's eastern Teso region. Her education came to an abrupt end when her father passed on while she was in Senior Three. Her widowed mother struggled to care for the large family, but when the bills to educate so many children became unbearable, Immaculate felt no option but to get married. She was happily living with her husband until she started falling sick. She had abdominal pain, constipation, and blood-stained stools, and a diagnosis of colorectal cancer came to her with much sadness.

Immaculate's condition was, however, especially worrying for her because she was almost eight months pregnant at the time the terrible news of her cancer diagnosis was revealed to her. 'This blow marked the beginning of my distress,' she narrated. In quick succession after learning that she had a serious tumour, her husband not only abandoned her but also sent her out of her matrimonial home, calling her a 'corpse' and proclaiming her end was near.

Immaculate returned to her mother's house and started to live with an elderly lady who was already poor and could hardly afford the transport fare to the nearest health facility.

Immaculate's health deteriorated very rapidly. Unable to bear any more the severe pain she was experiencing and the rectal bleeding which was draining her, Immaculate borrowed money from friends and neighbours and gathered just enough for the bus fare to bring her to the Uganda Cancer Institute at Mulago in Kampala.

It was while Immaculate was at the Cancer Institute that HAU was first called in to intervene. She urgently needed the care to control her overwhelming pain and symptoms. We enrolled her in our palliative care programme in January 2019. Immaculate gave birth a month later by caesarian section at Mulago Hospital to a bouncing baby boy. She named him Emmanuel, which means 'God with us' because she asserted that God never left her.

When she was discharged from the ward, Immaculate had nowhere to go with her son. Her home in Amuria was hundreds of miles away! She, therefore, made the difficult decision to spend the next several days with her baby living on the verandahs of the hospital floors. She and her baby were brought to the nearby hostel where patients temporarily live while undergoing treatment.

Immaculate was started on cancer chemotherapy, marking a rather new and tough chapter in her life. She was stopped from breastfeeding her one-month-old baby because of the risk that some of the chemotherapy medications could seep into her breastmilk and endanger the baby. Immaculate was between a rock and a hard place because not only was her health on the line but the very livelihood of her infant son was being taken away!

She had no support from home, she could hardly take care of herself and now she needed milk for the survival of her boy.

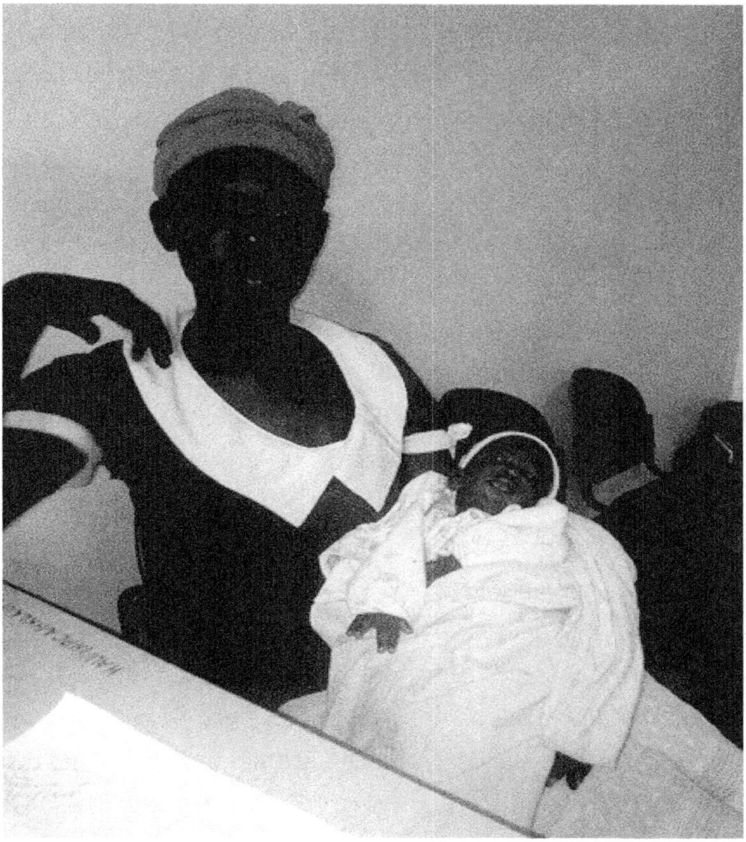

Photo 26: Immaculate with baby Emmanuel a few weeks after his birth

At this point Immaculate carried her two-month-old baby and took to Kampala streets to start begging, but this plan, hatched in desperation, failed because she was too weak to walk after receiving treatment. HAU intervened yet again. Immaculate appealed to Hospice to take care of her baby while she received treatment. We, in faith, agreed to this proposal.

Hospice continued offering palliative care services to Immaculate, then also mobilized resources for Baby Emmanuel to have a reliable supply of milk and a stock of essential items like diapers. The next challenge for Immaculate was the time spent in the hospital for exams and chemotherapy. Immaculate was not allowed to be with and nurse her baby during treatment and a crowded ward is far from an ideal place for an infant to live. HAU's social worker needed to think outside the box for this rather unusual situation. She approached the Kampala City Council Probation office with the uncommon request that they take on and settle the baby at a babies' home while his mother got treatment, rested, and recuperated.

Over several months, Immaculate attended the weekly daycare (when patients and caregivers come together for socialization and lunch) at HAU where she interacted with other patients and inspired many with the story of the challenges she was surmounting. Her visits to the daycare programme gave her a break from the monotony of the hospital ward.

For nearly two years, Immaculate had her treatments and her health improved. She also had surgery and a colostomy to relieve the agony of toileting with a colorectal tumour. Hospice ensures she always has a supply of colostomy bags.

She did not need to stay in hospital and the time of her discharge came. Attempts to reach her husband for support were futile. She needed to return to her village in Amuria district. HAU's social worker supplied the bus fare and coordinated with Immaculate's family back home to receive her. It was a joyous occasion when Immaculate reunited with her mother and siblings, and it was a wonderful homecoming with Emmanuel, now a toddler.

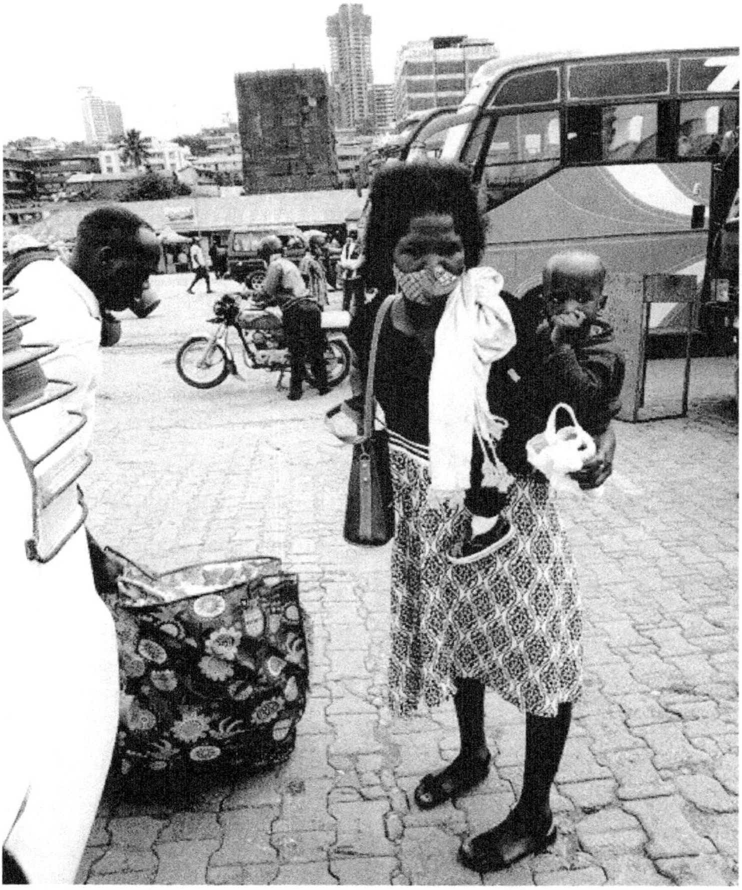

Photo 27: Immaculate and son Emmanuel waiting to board the bus to return home to her family

18

A Hand Up Rather than a Hand-out Made the Difference

Eddie Mwebesa and Roselight Katusabe

'Cate' is a 38-year-old lady, who was diagnosed with breast cancer at Mulago Hospital. She had surgery to remove her affected breast and thereafter went through many courses of radiotherapy and cycles of chemotherapy.

When she was enrolled in the palliative care programme at HAU in 2017, Cate had severe chest pain and a painful and swollen left arm. She was unable to carry out any activity and was dependent on others for her activities of daily living like bathing and dressing. The oral liquid morphine along with other medications Hospice gave her, were most helpful for the control of her severe pain and relief of the symptoms which were distressing her.

Although the physical pain Cate was experiencing was a prominent part of her existence when she first came to the Hospice, she also had marked psychosocial distress. She could no longer afford to sustain her children in school to receive basic education because when she fell sick, she depleted all her savings in the pursuit of life-sustaining treatments. HAU found Cate at a time when in addition to essential medicines to control her illnesses and the concurrent pain she suffered, she was also in dire need of social and financial support.

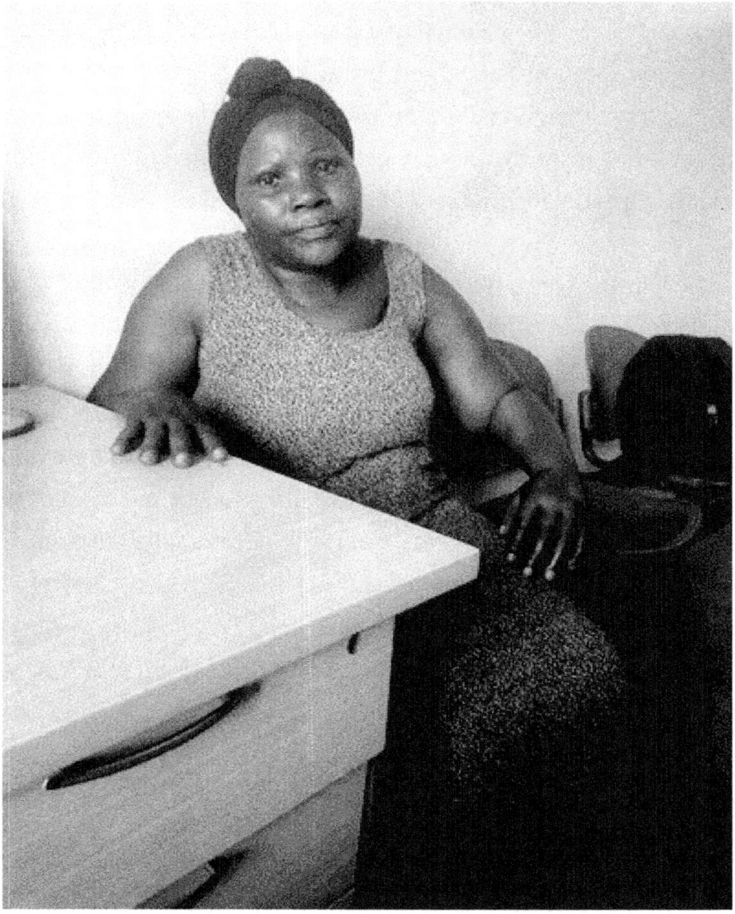

Photo 28: Cate at an earlier visit to the Hospice

As a charity, HAU is always bursting at the seams with more requests from suffering patients and their families than what our severely limited organizational budget can support. As the saying goes, 'Hospice is a friend' and Hospice has plenty of friends. We were motivated to mobilize and offer Cate resources of a livelihood nature because Hospice had assessed this patient and found that she had been a hard-working lady and very entrepreneurial. We reasoned that a hand-up would likely change around her circumstances and bring her to a place where she could sustain herself and her family.

HAU, therefore, wrote up Cate's story and shared it with our partners abroad. Our friends in Germany raised funds to support Cate.

The family was offered guidance and support by the HAU social worker and an assessment for the best use of the money was conducted. It became apparent that any physical work which personally involved Cate was not a great option. Cate, therefore, asserted that the best option was for her to procure a motorcycle and employ someone to ride it and return to her at the end of every day an income for daily domestic needs and a portion of the proceeds to be saved as tuition fees for her children's education.

Cate has gained the experience to manage this small business well and it has been profitable to date. Her health is good. She remains truly grateful to HAU and our friends abroad for the hand-up she received.

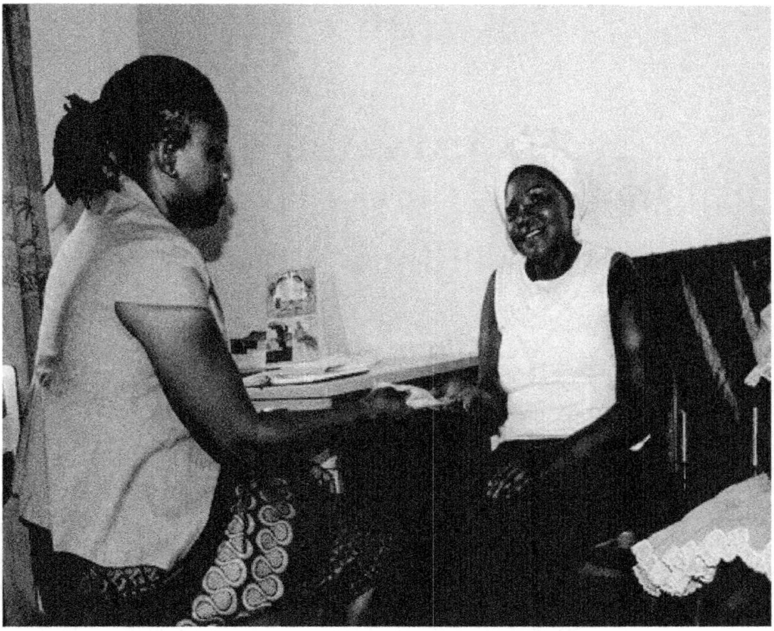

Photo 29: HAU's social worker handing over money to Cate for the start of her small business

19

A Typical Extra Mile Care by a Palliative Care Nurse to the Vulnerable during Covid

Roselight Katusabe

Working as a palliative care nurse during the era of the monster COVID-19 is quite scary and challenging! This is a time where a palliative care nurse must brave the worries and challenges associated with supporting vulnerable patients with palliative care needs under the limited availability of personal protective equipment against exposure to the virus.

Given the economic breakdown in the whole world, which is even worse in low-income countries including Uganda, our patients cannot afford transport to reach the facility and food to put in their stomachs; thus most of them are living in agony in communities near and far.

As a devoted and passionate palliative care nurse, I have gone the extra mile and visited these patients with the support of HAU, partner organizations like Road to Care (RTC), and individual well-wishers. These patients have varied needs ranging from food, medication, and access to health facilities like the Uganda Cancer Institute (UCI).

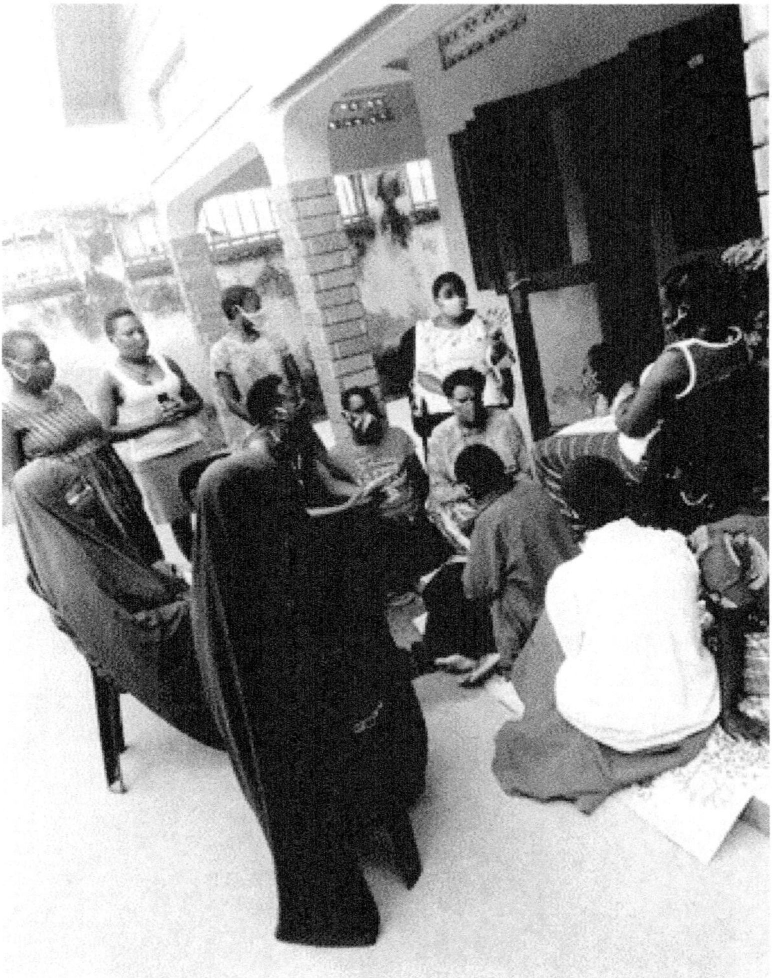

Photo 30: Meeting with cervical cancer patients at Uganda Cancer Institute

I and other HAU palliative care nurses have spent time sensitizing, counselling, and supporting patients with cervical cancer that have come to UCI for treatment, many with a lot of fears that they will get COVID-19. Some of their caretakers abandoned them in the Road to Care hostel and went back home in fear of being exposed to COVID-19. The majority of patients come with long-time vaginal bleeding due to inability to access health facilities which caused severe anaemia.

The government of Uganda also supported us by donating food that we have shared with the patients according to the severity of their needs. We have been able to sensitize the patients and their caretakers on how to prevent exposure to COVID-19 and teach them the dangers and complications of the virus and related after-effects.

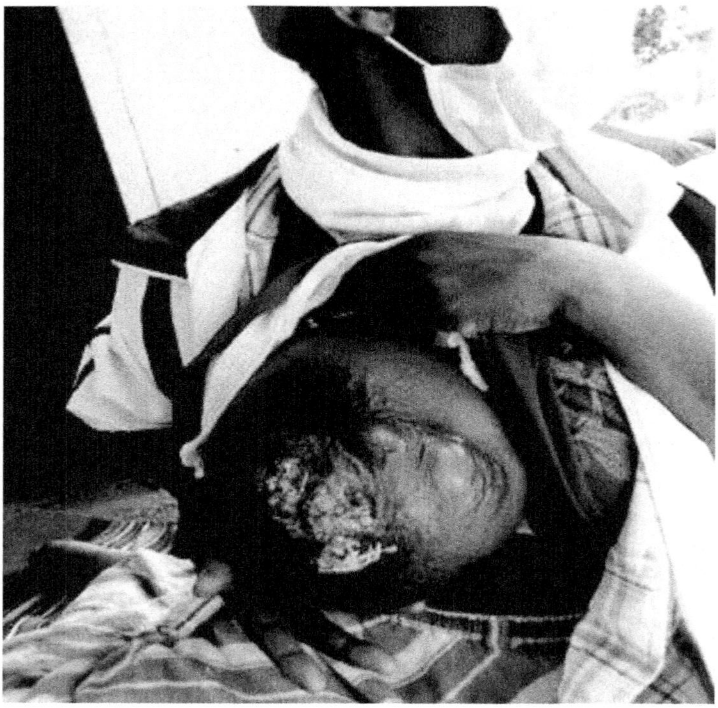

Photo 31: A patient with advanced breast cancer

We treat patients such as Zelda, who is 52 years old with advanced breast cancer. She has a touching story of episodes of sudden severe bleeding at home after failing to get radiotherapy due to lack of money to pay for the service. She has no physical carer so without HAU's support and a home visit, getting her pain and wound care medication would be next to impossible.

As a palliative care nurse and advocate who is a long-time advocate for Universal Health Coverage for all Uganda, I appeal to all well-wishers to further support HAU to get funding to help vulnerable patients access health facilities for early diagnosis and treatment. One of our models of service delivery is home-based care to the patients that are not able to come to the Hospice for outpatient review or are too sick to benefit from curative treatment in the hospital. The support will also help HAU to support patients with these basic needs as assessed.

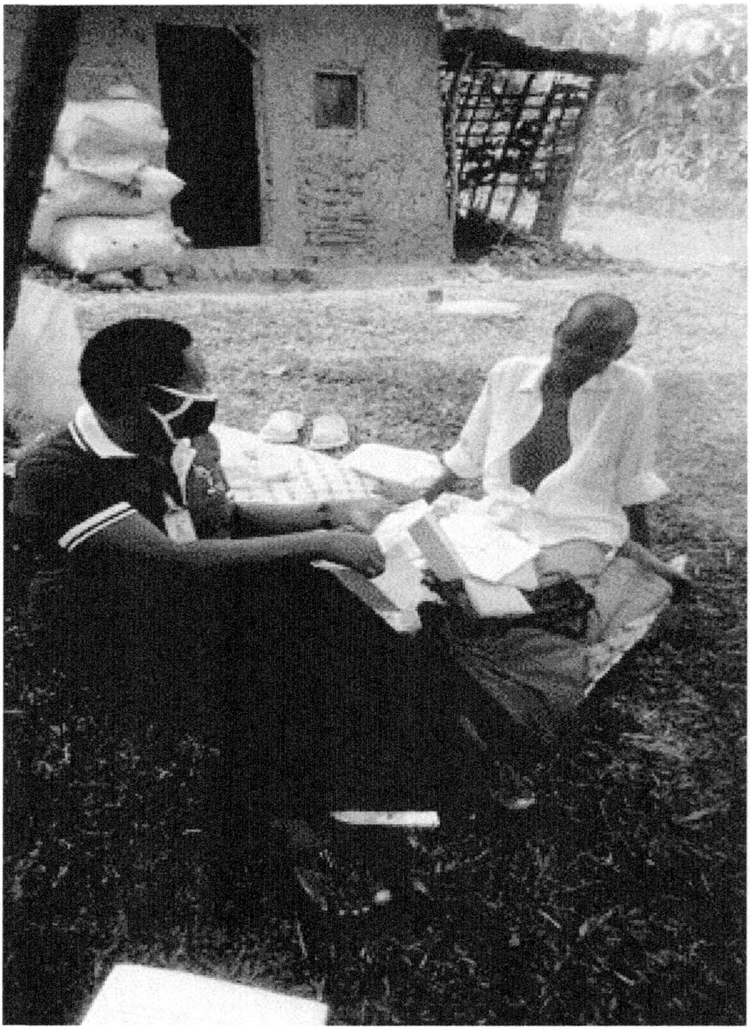

Photo 32: Roselight on a home visit to one of the most vulnerable patients. This was an 'extra mile' because he is outside the HAU catchment area

20

Dr Anne Merriman and the Birth of Hospice Africa

Successes and Challenges

Natuhwera Germans

Dr Anne Merriman is the founder of Hospice Africa Uganda (HAU), which has provided affordable, accessible, and culturally acceptable palliative care for patients with cancer, HIV, and other chronic conditions since 1993. In 1998, Dr Anne expanded HAU's reach by founding Mobile Hospice Mbarara; in later the same year, she opened a third site, Little Hospice Hoima.

She is known for her pioneering work, advocacy, and influential research in palliative care in low-resourced countries. Dr Merriman (known to all as Dr Anne) has pioneered and supported palliative care initiatives in SE Asia (Mlaywia and Singapore and across Africa: in Tanzania, Nigeria, Cameroon, Sierra Leone, Malawi, Ethiopia, Zambia, Sudan, Rwanda, and elsewhere. In addition to providing patient care, HAU operates the Institute of Hospice and Palliative Care in Africa, providing palliative care diploma and degree programmes for health care providers in Uganda and throughout Africa.

From HAU, the Palliative Care Association of Uganda (PCAU), an umbrella body for palliative care services in Uganda, was born, with Dr Anne as the founding Vice President. PCAU and HAU maintain close ties, both championing expansion of palliative care training, research, and availability to Ugandans in need.

Dr Anne continues to be motivated by exceptional compassionate love for patients, the vulnerable, and alleviation of suffering caused by cancer and other chronic illnesses. Those who have witnessed her extraordinary commitment are not surprised that at 88 years, Dr Anne still actively fundraises around the world to sustain the three Hospices, which depend largely on external donor funding. Her enthusiasm to keep sewing the seed of pain relief in Africa is incredible.

Natuhwera Germans recently had a dialogue with Prof. Merriman as she shared her story of pioneering palliative care in Africa.

Germans: *Reflecting back on the early days of introducing palliative care in Uganda, and Africa at large, what inspired you?*

Dr Anne: Hospice Africa was inspired by the suffering I witnessed in Nigeria in the 60s and in Kenya when working with Nairobi Hospice. The vision is '*Palliative care for all in need in Africa*'. The method we would use was planned in Liverpool where the first Board, Hospice Africa UK, commenced.

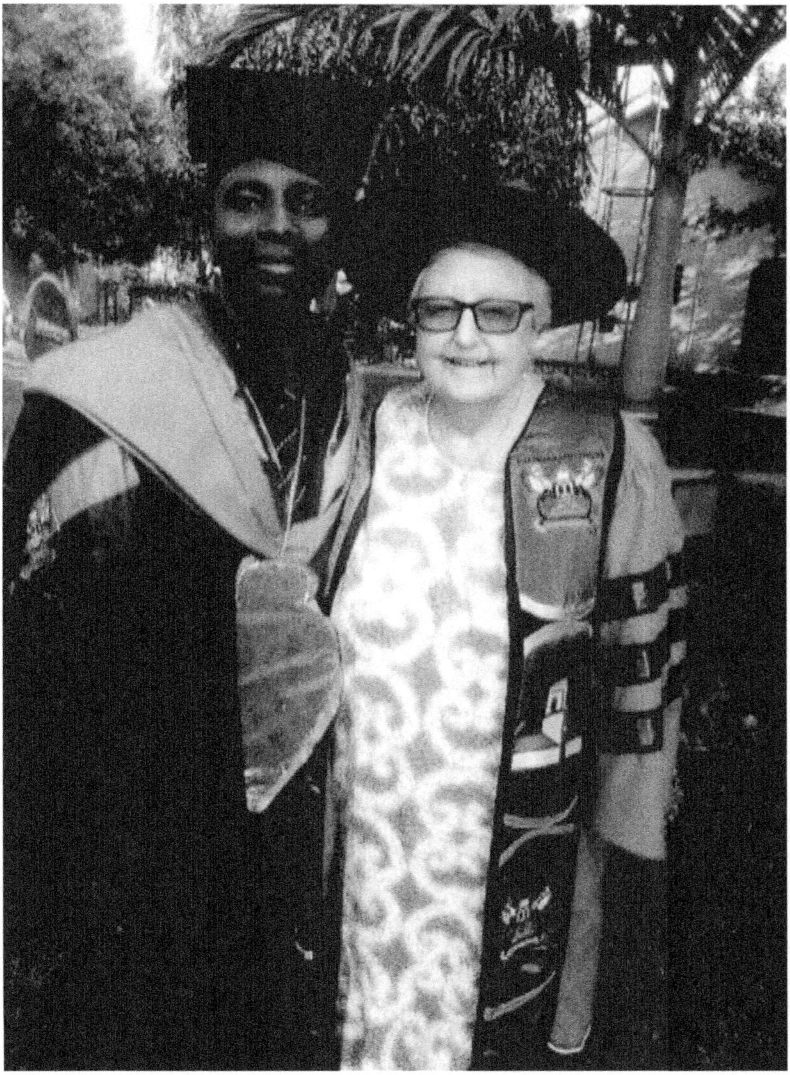

Photo 33: Natuhwera Germans and Dr Anne Merriman

Seven countries asked me to help them start services such as we had in Nairobi, following my article in the Christian journal *Contact* in 1992. We visited four countries to decide where to initiate the model. We chose Uganda because we needed a country with a good reputation with donors. Uganda was the best at the time as Museveni had done such a great job bringing Uganda out of war. He was at that time a darling of donors to Africa. Furthermore, Uganda had the lowest corruption estimate of the four finalist we seriously considered.

The country was poor and just coming out of war and needed support for cancer, as HIV was already receiving a lot of funding. HIV was rampant and had doubled the incidence of cancer.

When the then Minister of Health, Dr James Makumbi, heard of the oral affordable morphine we had designed and used in Singapore and Kenya successfully without any addiction said, 'My people are suffering, please come…'.

Germans: *What are you happy/unhappy about with regards to palliative care in Uganda/Africa? What opportunities and challenges have you faced, and remain for palliative care?*

Dr Anne: I'm happy about the support from Uganda's Ministry of Health from 1998 to 2004. Following a conference bringing together all those involved with suffering, a committee was formed and chaired by Dr Jack Jagwe. It took a long time for their appeal for a change in the statute allowing midwives to prescribe pethidine (a pain-relieving opioid) to be expanded so that nurses specially trained in palliative care and registered could also prescribe. Up to then only doctors, vets and dentists could prescribe and we had (and still have) so few doctors that there are not enough to see, assess, and prescribe for the thousands in pain.

In 2003, the statute was passed and the Diploma in Clinical Palliative Care commenced at HAU. Also since then, our Government has paid for morphine production so that oral morphine is free to all in severe pain who are prescribed by a recognized prescriber, on the PCAU list of prescribers.

On challenges, I'm particularly dissatisfied by the lack of recognition of palliative care as a specialty. It has been a specialty in the UK since 1986, in the US since 2006 and now in several African countries but not Uganda. I am also disappointed in the lack of knowledge on the extent of palliative care available in the country by those making public health decisions.

Now with Covid-19, patients need palliative care more than ever. Palliative care has the answer to breathlessness and pain that is a large part of the suffering and supports the existential suffering which comes with unexpected approach of death. The failure of other specialities to call us in early enough to know the patients and family before the end is a challenge as well – this is improving, but slowly.

Germans: *Where do you see HAU and palliative care in the next ten years? Funding? Sustainability of the service...?*

Dr Anne: Palliative care is here to stay. Uganda is still seen as having the best palliative care in Africa, but others are taking over this as they are now coming up fast. Oral affordable morphine has increased. African countries with palliative care have gone from three in 1993 when HAU commenced to 37 through our training and the advocacy to change ancient policies and myths regarding addiction.

It is through training that the vision for palliative care across Africa will be met in years to come. This is through the Institute of Hospice and PC in Africa (IHPCA) and our department of International Programmes that bring students for clinical training here twice a year from Anglo and Francophone countries. With the support of PCAU in 1999, which bring us all together, palliative care has expanded from one district to 107 throughout Uganda.

The African Palliative Care Association (APCA) brings all the African countries together and advocates internationally to African governments as well as other areas. Funding is now scarce, and Covid-19 has made matters worse. Many of our patients are poor and living below the poverty line and now are hungry also, so food is a big problem.

At our best we cared for between 1,500 patients and 2,000 at any one time, but now up to 700 only because of the reduction in donors who are now supporting the many other tragedies in this world. But the need for pain control and reduction of suffering night and day is very real and we still need assistance at double the present assistance, regularly.

Germans: *Any other things to mention, recommendations to stakeholders, civil society organizations, media, government, private sector...?*

Dr Anne: External donors are reducing, and unless Uganda can carry us forward with funding, palliative care will fail. We must remember that none of us will live forever. We cannot take our money with us. Let us use it for the needy now. These are our brothers and sisters, whether rich or poor. Palliative care is needed by us all when our turn comes, to relieve the pain and symptoms and to assist with support for you and your family.

Martha Rabwoni is a specialist palliative care nurse and the Health Services Coordinator at Mobile Hospice Mbarara. She is one of the first two nurses who worked with Prof. Merriman to start up HAU in Uganda in the very early days and has worked with HAU since 1993 to date. Martha describes Dr Anne in these words:

'Dr Anne is focused and if she wants anything she has to get it no matter what. She's very compassionate, and she's someone who values everyone; that is what has kept Hospice going for all these years. Anne makes her vision known to everyone she's working with ... I think Anne has done her part. The rest is ours to make sure that her legacy lives on when she's no longer here. We can't hold onto her forever, she's a human being.'

21

A Life of Caring and Teaching

Meet the Third Nurse to Join Dr Anne at HAU

Racheal Dipio

I was always eager to pursue a career where my job would be to support those who are unable to care and fend for themselves. As a child, I loved helping vulnerable people; and at the age of 12 years, I joined the Adjumani Catholic Parish youth group called the Crusaders. The Crusaders had a similar function to the Banna Kizito of Kampala Archdioceses. They would go in the villages to help the poor, the sick, and the elderly with house chores, taking them food and cleaning their household surroundings.

My coming to HAU was a calling from God! In February 1995, while working with Nsambya Hospital, we were informed that HAU wanted to train a nurse in palliative care for the hospital. The first nurse identified for the training declined the offer, and I was given the chance to go for the training. When I shared the news with my colleagues, many discouraged me, based on their perception that HAU only cares for the dying. Nevertheless, I accepted the offer and saw it as an opportunity to escape the hospital night duties that interfered with my young family.

In March 1995, I joined HAU as a Registered Nurse not sure of what I was heading for. I learned to appreciate its informality, quite different from hospital setting, where hierarchical norms were not strictly observed and adhered to. The small HAU family was so welcoming; I was particularly surprised by the 'relaxed' atmosphere: Staff did not wear uniforms, and staff and volunteers were called by their names to give a more informal feeling to patients and their families. As a calm, quiet and task-oriented person, I blended very well with the HAU team.

The HAU environment helped me to overcome the bereavement process I was going through having lost my first-born four months earlier. I shall forever be indebted to the team for their immeasurable support during this time. The experience I had at HAU was quite contrary to the perception my friends had about working there; being in a palliative care organization helped in quickening my healing process.

When I joined HAU, it only had a team of eight members. With a small team, HAU prioritized induction of health professionals as a key priority. In her role as HAU's founder and director, Dr Anne taught and encouraged the members of staff, especially when reviewing patients. This training laid a firm foundation for my clinical skills. These inductions were followed by mentorship and coaching by the senior HAU nurses, Rose Kiwanuka and Martha Rabwoni, who had been with Dr Anne from the beginning.

In 1998, two additional branches of HAU were established – Mobile Hospice Mbarara (MHM) and Little Hospice Hoima (LHH). This led to transfer of the senior staff to manage the newly established branches. We remaining staff members had the challenge of taking on new leadership roles. I was appointed

Health Services Coordinator to lead the clinical team, a position I held for six years.

Palliative care nursing is challenging, demanding, and rewarding. Pursuing a career in palliative medicine is all about compassion, courage, communication, competence, care, and commitment. I can confidently say I have these values and skills, and I believe I have made a difference in the lives of people I assisted and their families during their difficult times.

Relief of patients' pain and symptoms always inspired me at HAU. Seeing a patient who came in pain able to smile, removing the terrible fungating (ulcerating) wound odour by cleaning and application of metronidazole powder, and just being there for a patient and family, listening to their issues was a heart touching and a learning experience.

One day, while on a home visit in Kawempe, I came across a patient who was terribly disfigured; one could hardly identify the face. He was abandoned by his relatives in a small room with severe pain and was helpless. Seeing this patient broke my heart. I made a promise that wherever there is a very ill patient within our reach, he/she will be taken care of in the best way possible. Patients and family came first; the team always endeavoured to visit patients even late in the afternoon in cases of emergencies. Night calls were received by Dr Anne and those who called HAU were received by a guard (day/night) and the teams were informed for action.

In 2000, funding was secured from donors and a new building was constructed and named 'Rutamwebwa House'. The Clinical and Education departments moved to this building, which had spacious working environment and improved privacy for patients. The Merriman Lounge remained for daycare and administration. We shared experiential clinical teaching to medical students from Makerere University and other universities including international students. We also received some international volunteer doctors for placement.

Home-based care has been HAU's unique practical learning resource, including caring for patients referred from other hospitals around Kampala, many from Mulago National Referral Hospital. Accompanying us on home-based visits enabled students to experience the holistic aspect of our care. The interaction with students, volunteers, and various visitors enabled not only sharing of knowledge but they also learnt the ethos that they were able to take back to their facilities. Other clinical learning took place in case conferences and journal clubs.

Having worked as Health Services Coordinator, I also had the opportunity to further my education and career. I took the initiative to undertake a Diploma in Palliative Care and Diploma in Clinical Palliative Care, in addition to other relevant undergraduate and postgraduate courses. I also had work experience placement in Reach out Mbuya HIV/AIDS Initiative and Mildmay Uganda, where I was given the opportunity to shadow doctors and nurses.

In August 2004, I was transferred to HAU's Distance Learning Department (DLD), which was running a Diploma in Palliative Care course affiliated with Makerere University. In addition, I participated in the HAU's district programme that promoted the integration of palliative care in the District HIV/AIDS care activities in Uganda.

The Education department also conducted short courses in Clinical Palliative Care and a Diploma in Clinical Palliative Care (DCPC), which commenced at the same time with DLD programme in 2002. In 2011, the two departments were merged and evolved into 'Institute of Hospice and Palliative Care in Africa' (IHPCA), which offers short courses, diploma, undergraduate, and postgraduate programmes in palliative care. The Institute's undergraduate and later postgraduate courses were affiliated with Makerere University.

Under the International Programme, I participated in training/mentoring students in the following countries: Ethiopia, Malawi, Sudan, and Tanzania. This exposure widened my knowledge in palliative care. Since 2011, I have worked as a Lecturer at IHPCA with a talented, zealous, and committed team. The joy of witnessing this growth of HAU is like watching your beloved baby grow into a mature person. Many students have passed through my hand through formal classroom teaching as well as clinical teaching, as our patients are our teacher.

Palliative care nurses need to pay attention to details that would enable them notice any changes in the condition of the patient. The ability to keep calm under difficult and intense pressure is an essential skill for nurses. I developed these skills while taking part in managing USAID funds to implement short courses, prepare activity reports and accounting for funds spent. I also learnt the initiative of resolving situations related to patient needs and ensuring the best possible outcome for individual patients.

No day of work at HAU was the same. I met different people, with different needs, and under different conditions. At times, things did not go as planned; you had to be ready, thinking on your feet to solve an emerging situation while remaining calm. As a palliative care nurse, I learnt new things every day from my colleagues and patients, which inspired me to explore deeper knowledge on the best techniques and procedures.

The goal of Hospice is to improve quality of life of patients in their last months, focusing on comfort care, control of pain, and symptom management, as opposed to continuing curative treatments. However, palliative care can commence right from the time of diagnosis until the end of life. Regardless of the stage at which patients enter the programme, efforts should be concentrated on improving their quality of life.

Palliative care is important for cancer patients who are able to afford disease-modifying treatment like chemotherapy and/or radiation or even surgery as a curative treatment. While this treatment is often effective at shrinking, destroying, or removing cancer cells, it has a wide range of side effects including nausea, loss of appetite, skin burns, dry mouth, fatigue, and constipation. Addressing these side effects improves the patient's overall quality of life, which is why palliative care should be considered whenever a patient receives a diagnosis of serious or chronic illness.

Many patients pass on in hospitals because they are unable to afford disease-modifying treatment, yet as the disease advances pain and other symptoms also increase, requiring palliative care. Other patients go to hospitals early enough, but investigations take too long, giving chance for the disease to advance. In these situations, the only option left is palliative care, where pain and distressing symptoms are controlled to improving the quality of life of the patient. Conversely, some patients go to hospitals when the disease is quite advanced. Without palliative care, hospitalized patients at the end of life often receive inconsistent care and during their final wishes, relatives or families are not involved. Through its holistic approach, HAU offers patients and their families the opportunity to spend their final days together in a compassionate environment, with the aim of making them as comfortable as possible.

In my years of working as a nurse at HAU, I noted that seriously ill patients understand the value of each passing day. While facing their illness, the support of palliative care in controlling pain and other distressing symptoms can make each day a more positive experience and allows the patient to make the most of the time they have left with their families.

Working in HAU has enriched my life spiritually. I see the work of God in whatever I do and call upon Him daily for wisdom and strength. It has also enabled me realize the humanity in me, hence helping others. In my opinion and experience, nurses unknowingly gain more resilience in handling their challenges as they interact with patients and families. For instance, whenever something bad happens, I focus on the positive side, believing that everything happens for a reason. This was not the case before I joined HAU.

22

Reflections on My Path in Palliative Care Nursing at Hospice Africa Uganda

Bernadette Mandera

As I reflect back on my path in palliative care, one word defines my journey – perseverance. Whether in my personal or professional life, I have faced critical situations that required a high level of focus, hard work, and maturity to resolve the situation. These experiences have enabled me take up various positions at HAU. I have served as Senior Nurse, Assistant Health Services Coordinator, and carried out teaching and training in palliative care. I also was a teaching assistant and later Associate Lecturer at the Institute of Hospice and Palliative Care in Africa (IHPCA). My personal values along with my other skills and experiences enabled me to be a successful nurse at HAU.

I began my nursing career with an interest in science and business. All along, I wanted to be involved in caring, but my sponsor suggested I take up a teaching career. I objected because my father was a teacher and he used to stay up very late preparing lesson plans, which didn't appeal to me. I eventually chose a nursing career and joined nursing school to realize my dreams.

Unexpectedly, my dad passed on as the result of an accident when I had just qualified as a Registered Nurse in 1993. Six years later, my mother also passed on in April 1999 because of liver disease. This happened a year after I had joined HAU and brought to light the importance of palliative care and the need for monitoring one's health. My parents' deaths serve as a painful reminder of the human element involved in palliative care, one that I take with me each day. Despite the emotional and physical difficulties I experienced, life had to continue. I resumed work with a new drive to attain a career in palliative care, where I used my experience and compassion to keep the patient's voice strong and increased access to quality care.

In 2002, I obtained a Diploma in Clinical Palliative Care, and was immediately appointed a Senior Nurse and Assistant Health Service Coordinator in the Clinical Department. I was later transferred to the Education Department in 2006, which is now IHPCA.

I have worked in IHPCA for 15 years and have done plenty of teaching, a career I thought I had avoided. Although, good in clinical teaching, I had minimal knowledge of palliative care classroom teaching; nonetheless, I was determined, I pushed myself hard to learn and eventually I succeeded. My career development as a palliative care nurse continued until I obtained Diploma in Palliative Care from Makerere University in 2005 and thereafter was promoted to a position of Palliative Care Trainer in 2005. In 2011, I became a Teaching Assistant at IHPCA and later as an Associate Lecturer. In 2013, I graduated with a Bachelors of Palliative Care degree from Makerere

University and currently I am pursuing Post Graduate Diploma in Palliative Care (PGDPC).

Working as Palliative Care Trainer encompassed all I had mastered as an Assistant Health Services Coordinator and Senior Nurse. It required looking at the Clinical Department from an overall outpatient-home based care facility perspective. Although these positions were challenging, it gave me an opportunity to experience the daily struggles and successes associated with managing a department, while developing my leadership skills.

When I arrived at HAU, my first patient was a woman with advanced ovarian cancer. She had a grossly distended abdomen, severe wasting, protruding eyes, and a sick look that worried me at first sight. Although I came from a hospital setting, I had never come across such a disturbing condition. I felt very sad and sorry for the patient and her two little children aged four and six years old.

The senior nurse with whom I had gone quickly realized that I was saddened. She encouraged me by telling me that the patient was pain free although she had abdominal discomfort. We agreed to ask the doctor if tapping (taking off fluid) could help and at this point, I had a bit of relief. We cleaned the patient after counselling, put her in upright position and encouraged the caregiver. The patient had barely anything to eat. We arranged to provide a weekly food supply from HAU's Comfort Fund.

Despite her advanced disease and lack of food, the care of her two little girls was the dying mother's main distress. This situation made me realize that palliative care nursing in the hospital mainly entails providing interventions to handle the disease, while home-based palliative care nursing plays a broader role: prevention and reduction of patient suffering through management of physical symptoms along with provision of psychosocial and spiritual support for the patient.

In my early years, many patients sick with HIV/AIDS reported to HAU with limited anti-retroviral medications (ARVs). Only a few patients could afford the high costs of chemotherapy/radiotherapy or even surgery as required by the diagnosis/stage and sensitivity to the treatment. We looked after many patients and lost quite a number of them who were emotionally drained because they were referred either too late or reported late to hospitals due to various reasons like poverty, lack of knowledge about their illnesses, trial of herbal medicines, long distances to hospitals, and availability of the required services.

Yet we were comforted that the majority, died pain free and their symptoms were improved. We were able to achieve this through teamwork; the team member's focus was on the patient and family care. This value was reinforced by the HAU spirit of '*love and care for one another*' which we encouraged and practised.

My expertise in palliative care nursing did not depend only on classroom teaching; much of it came from home care visits, case conferences, journal clubs and team discussions. We had several local and international senior doctors and nurses who were enthusiastic in teaching and providing support. We also received visitors and students from the African sub-region and other countries, with whom we taught, shared experiences, and improved palliative care teaching.

The extraordinary passion for stewardship, patient-centred care, and perseverance enabled me to succeed as a palliative care nurse. My main contribution to HAU service took place between

2004 and 2008, when I helped lead Comprehensive District Training Programmes in Mukono, Arua, and Gulu Districts. These programmes required an understanding of not only classroom teaching but also clinical and administrative support, teamwork, and collaboration to operate efficiently while providing quality palliative care.

Caring for those with advanced cancer or other life-threatening illness requires compassion and love in taking care of the physical, psychosocial, and spiritual needs to reduce the patient's suffering for a more dignified death. This approach also improves the quality of life of caregivers, who invest a lot of time and energy taking care of terminally ill patients. The courage and dedication to fulfilling the complex needs of a dying patient became a unique experience for me as a palliative care nurse. Powerful and complex emotions often emerge as patients with life-limiting illnesses approach their end of life. Helping them gain spiritual peace is a very important aspect of palliative care.

As I wrote this recollection of my time at HAU, I kept posing questions to myself as to whether what happened over these years of work was meant to test my ability or faith as a palliative care nurse. I also keep wondering whether I would be alive if I had not become a palliative care nurse. Palliative care knowledge has helped and is still helping me, especially in managing my own distressing symptoms because sometimes I get emotionally overwhelmed. Palliative care has improved my quality of life and that of my family significantly. When I think of the patients without access to palliative care, I surely share their pain and appreciate the troubling experience they are going through.

My journey at HAU was marked with challenges and uncertainty. I met each one with determination and willingness to work and kept at it until they were addressed. I encourage the young doctors, nurses, and all who care for patients to take appropriate approaches to the challenges they will face as they continue to develop their careers and leadership skills in palliative care and promote the mission of HAU.

I wish every health professional had the interest and opportunity to care for patients with life limiting illness. The rewards for this noble course of work are beyond counting.

Finally, I wish to appreciate the work done by Dr Anne Merriman, the founder and first CEO of HAU. She laid a firm foundation that has kept HAU fulfilling its role of providing palliative care training and services to Ugandans. In the same breath, I would like to acknowledge the support given to HAU and in particular, to IHPCA, by the Government of Uganda, development partners, funding agencies, and well-wishers.

23

Uniqueness in Everyone

Personalizing Care

Francisca Nagujja

End of life care has no formula as each family holds its own beliefs, culture, and perspectives, not to mention the attending clinicians. The reactions family members give once the clinician informs them their dear one is dying varies. Some will cry, others may react with silence; some will take it positively while others will deny what has been said.

As a palliative care nurse, most of the patients I encounter are in their final journey on Earth, but this journey differs in both the time they have and how they respond to the information that they are nearing the end of their lives. For example, we know that most patients with cancer of the oesophagus will spend six months to a year in palliative care before dying; this gives us good time to prepare. There are others who you may think are dying soon and who surprisingly live longer. As a health worker, I have learnt never to say how long someone must live, even when I know he or she is dying today. I will only tell the family that the patient is dying, in order to avoid commotions and mistrust in the care we give. Once we give them an eye opener that your patient is dying, they are usually able to digest that patient likely has one month or less to live.

I remember around 2015 we received a lady with advanced disease from a brain tumour who was discharged from hospital for end-of-life care. Surprisingly even on the referral note the doctor had specified end-of-life care, not palliative care, unlike what most clinicians list. She was in a vegetative state with a dismantled family following a disruptive social history. She groaned with pain and presented with convulsions. It was such a trying moment for her twin daughters who had spent some good time without seeing the mother because of community and family misunderstandings. The patient was enrolled, and daughters counselled. They hoped she would die soon as she was so very ill, and asked how long it would be until she died.

On that day we had a visiting doctor from Europe who frankly told them six months. This prediction brought a debate among clinicians as to why the doctor had disclosed this. We explained that in African culture stating a specific time the patient will die is not good as it may raise issues among the family, patient and attending health care workers. The doctor boldly replied that, after all, that's what she had to live and jokingly we told her to come back after six months to witness what she had said.

We provided ongoing counselling to the daughters, advising them always to be present at home, talk good things to their mother, give her pain medications and others as prescribed, and allow her friends and religious leader to visit.

Guess what happened? In six months, the patient greatly improved; by the end of the year, she was able to go to the garden only sustained on anti-convulsant and pain medications. She lived two good years on palliative care. The day she died, her daughter reported that they both went to the garden, came back home, had lunch and she had taken a rest in the bed as always, since it was her routine, and she didn't wake up. That was the end. This taught me not to just look at the physical appearance of the patient or think she/he will die at a certain time.

I believe for all non-Africans, who routinely predict how long patients have to live, disclosing this may be tricky. However much you find the family strong enough to take the bad news, for those patients who exceed the time given most of the carers will lose trust and they may end up not coming back for care. Plus, we have learned that such predictions are often inaccurate – all the more reason to keep them to ourselves, or tell the family that this is God's time!

At Hospice Africa Uganda (HAU) and Mobile Hospice Mbarara (Hospice) we have four modes of service delivery: home-based, outpatient, hospital-based and outreach based. In all these services an important element is phone follow up. If you are the one on the other end of the phone patients use to contact clinicians, you have to be ready for anything.

I coordinate the bereavement programme and I've noticed that the last one to three days of patients' lives are the most terrible and worrying to the family, especially if the patient has distressing symptoms. Usually when a patient or family member calls during working hours the clinician has access to the patient's file to refer to. But no matter when a carer calls, you have to be present physically, psychologically, and spiritually. While callers ask about medications, review dates, or increasing pain/symptoms, they will also call to tell you their patient has died or is gasping with death rattle. I have encountered so many carers who call when the patient is dying at that very minute and I have to be ready to talk them through this difficult time.

I will never forget two similar scenarios of which I will narrate one. This lady had hepato-cellular carcinoma, with gross ascites (fluid build-up in the abdomen), which caused severe breathing distress. She was referred to Hospice in her final months. At the end of life since she had moved from one hospital to another bargaining that she would find a cure.

She was referred for palliative care by a friend who was a patient of the programme. We used to visit her home to care for her. She was Muslim, which often means many carers around a very sick person. The last home visit was two days before her death. As it was clear death was near, the clinician reported the situation to the team just in case we got a phone call. I was lucky (or unlucky) enough that I was on call the day she died.

I remember it was a Saturday night. I was watching a very good film, hoping for no distractions, and here came the patient phone call. It alarmed me – I could hear the panic among her carers. They had called a nearby doctor to do something; he simply told them to bring the patient to hospital. The one who called was angry and was counting on me to give a final verdict on whether to take the patient to hospital then or wait till morning and make a visit since the patient was nearby. Before saying anything, I remember telling him that I need the holy spirit; and indeed, the holy spirit intervened.

No, I didn't actually see the holy spirit, but given how I handled the case I couldn't believe it was me. I told the man to give the phone to the doctor. I could hear the patient 'grating,' meaning death rattle. I asked the doctor if the patient was calm in bed and indeed, she was except that noisy breathing. He also agreed that the patient was dying. In our discussion, he realized that taking patient to hospital was not necessary but that the goals should be to calm the family.

I told him to put me on speakerphone so that everyone could hear what I was saying. The good thing was that all her children, brothers and sisters were there, plus several friends. I told them the meaning of that sound and we all agreed on what the patient would like now. I remember asking one of her children to hold her hand and pat it, while others should say a prayer since she was a prayerful person. They elevated the bed as I asked. I told them that the patient may stay in this situation for some time but all we needed was to keep calm for her. I also told them that her ears were still functioning so our panicking would make her panic too. They did all that I asked, and everyone calmed down. I could hear the patient breathing calmly.

Only then did I disconnect the phone. This was one of the longest phone calls I have ever made. It was for over an hour, with the added challenge that I am not fluent in Runyakore, the native language. No sooner had I resumed my movie than I received another phone call thanking me for the good last moment they had with their mother. Death happened 20 minutes after our talk.

Some may wonder how we do it. All I can say you don't have to be experienced in end-of-life counselling, but you do have to be prepared all the time that patients and family will walk in or call and be in immediate need of this vital support. Being present all the time even when you have a thousand thoughts because you're knowing someone beloved by their family is dying anytime can't be equated to the usual problems. It's like losing a precious diamond or your mother's precious gift. It exposes you to knowing that death is real and all the time we must be ready for it. It doesn't matter how close or how related you are to the patient and carers; your job in that moment is giving them the feeling that they have someone to rely on who can relate to the way they are feeling at that time.

During my general training I never took death that seriously and rarely did I encounter people dying. Most of my experience was sudden deaths which didn't allow for counselling, or clinicians had no confidence in providing this kind of support and it wasn't offered. Even the doctors would see patients dying and would tell the family, 'She is doing better; all will be well.'

I now feel strongly that patients and families are entitled to know how serious the situation may be. Patients will almost never bring up the topic of death and dying but as clinicians we must introduce death topics so that people are able to prepare and make adjustments or make decisions that will help their families once they are gone. My palliative care training opened my understanding of the many stages we have to appreciate as life is filled with steps of being born, living fully and then encountering death. The most important thing is having a peaceful death, which means different things to different people.

As a clinician, dying peacefully or a dignified death may mean being physically pain free. However other priorities count more for some people. For example, we may wonder why most patients with cancer of the oesophagus refuse a gastrostomy tube / feeding tube. Most I have encountered prefer dying with their bodies intact with no artificial implant. Since most of them are 60 and above they usually say 'I have lived my life. I have eaten enough; even when my disease doesn't allow me to eat, what else am I gaining in this world?'

Most elderly patients with gangrene who refuse amputation say, 'I was not born lame, why die with only one leg? Just control my pain, take away the smell and leave the rest to God.' And most of these patients who refuse intervention are discharged against doctors advise. You can only understand these patients if you have had a palliative care course. It used to frustrate me every time I met a dying patient who refused interventions at the time when they would help; but now I understand that from the patient's perspective they will not reverse anything.

Why am I bringing up this point about patients' differing ideas about peaceful dying? Because every time I am conducting end of life counselling, I know it's my job to find out what they mean by being peaceful. The recent patient I saw with cancer of the stomach told me, 'I am glad my children have completed school though they haven't gotten married.' So, his final wish was to see a wedding of any of his children and then he could rest. At the end of our session, he wished to be referred to Hospice before starting chemotherapy.

He left with peace of mind and, with his physical pain controlled, it made even things much better. These personal issues give you a guide on how to counsel patients through their remaining journey.

Even our mere presence is a medicine of its own, much as when I go for medical care, I feel satisfied when the attending doctor gives me his or her time, which very few do. For too many physicians, the time we give our patients is regarded as time wasting but for us palliative care practitioners, we feel satisfied and happy that at the end the one who was worried and scared leaves with hope that all will be well, even knowing the end may be near.

I remember during our fundraising we visited an Anglican church. One of the Christians asked if we were born again. To my understanding he regarded our work as a vocation. If you are not called to do it then you won't stay in it for long. I have seen those who come for a short while and leave without saying goodbye. Interns come and appreciate our work, but some fear seeing dying patients.

It is easy to console one who still has the innermost living. They will never mind what illness they have; the most important thing is that they are still breathing. We encounter so many patients with the inner spirit living yet the body is dismantled like a wrecked ship.

A recent memory is of a lady with advanced HCC (liver cancer). She was eight months on palliative care before she died. But slowly she was losing her weight to the point where she had only a skeletal body. All her body mass was gone, and she was left with the skin covering the internal organs. The family was poor, but declined interventions not out of lack of finances but because they didn't want their beloved mother to be tortured in any way.

We visited her in her little village every two weeks. End of life counselling wasn't applicable to her because she said, 'God gives life and when He decides He takes it away so am ready for anything. The only thing am grateful for is that He brought you into my house and now am pain free. I can laugh and converse with my children.' We counselled the children, and they came to terms with their mother's situation. She smiled all the time. She welcomed everyone, including the neighbours, and showed interested in each and every thing. I remember her saying, 'Even when I have bones alone my heart is still strong.' She appreciated every small thing and indeed the team misses her beautiful smile.

In her last days she said, 'I wish you would get me a small bun (round bread) and some sugar and I will feel satisfied enough to go.' It was she was saying bye-bye to us. The next visit was three days later. We brought her the bun and some milk. The children told us that she ate the things we gave her without any difficulty yet other days they would force her eat even a 50 mls cup of milk. She died two days after this. We were happy that we had met someone with a free and caring spirit; this gave us morale as a team to keep caring for those who had lost it.

Even with the challenges Hospice is facing, I believe the blessings that patients pray will make it last forever. We may have more intercedes up in heaven. I always pray that in case we the team need this kind of help someone will be there to guide us and our families. We can't thank enough the Almighty God who has given us opportunities to take care of such precious people. And for all the patients who passed on in our care, we are thankful that God grants them eternal rest. And may He show us the way in caring for those still searching for our help. Amen.

24

Breaking Bad News

My Personal Experience

Miriel Kabigarire

> Telling the truth is one of the most powerful therapeutic agents available to us but we still need to develop a proper understanding of its clinical pharmacology and to recognize optimum timing and dosage in its use.
>
> (Robert Twycross, 2003)

Before I joined palliative care, I regarded breaking bad news as sitting down with the patient and family to provide information about a diagnosis or poor prognosis. However, working as a palliative care nurse, I soon understood that breaking bad news is best seen as a process, not a one-off event. We must carefully consider how we share bad, sad, or difficult information that alters patients' and families' perceptions of their present and future.

If not done thoughtfully, communicating bad news, such as a malignant tumour or other life-threatening cancer, may also be invasive. The effects of bad communication with a patient can metastasize to the family and cause lasting harm and traumatic memories for all involved. I share a personal story to illustrate this fact.

I was the primary carer to my late mother who succumbed to death following hypertension complications. She was admitted in one of the biggest hospitals in Uganda due to a weak heart; her heart rate was low and she needed a pacemaker. The doctors told us the pacemaker had been ordered from South Africa and we needed to patiently wait. We spent three weeks on the ward waiting for the pacemaker delivery.

One evening, my mother's doctor announced to us that my mum's pacemaker had arrived and the next morning she was to be taken to the operating theatre to have it implanted. We were very happy that my mother was to be worked on and the next day we could finally take her home.

She was taken to theatre the next morning as the doctor had promised us. I remained at the theatre entrance waiting for my mum to come out from theatre as I had been told that pacemaker implantation was a short procedure. Two hours, then four and six hours passed and my mother was still not out. It wasn't until the eighth hour that the doctor called me into a room. I could read on his face that something was wrong. I asked him if there was anything wrong with my mother and he did not tell me. He only said that my mother had needed open heart surgery and that she was out of danger. This was a terrible shock; no one had even informed me that my mother was in surgery. And in my heart, I could not believe his words because he was looking unsure of what he was saying.

I fainted right then and there and found myself in a room surrounded by the theatre team trying to give me first aid. After recovering from the shock, still no one sat me down to explain what could have happened to my mum. It was late and everyone was going home. It wasn't until the eleventh hour, after almost no information from anyone, that I discovered myself that my mother had died.

The doctors plus the whole theatre team feared to break the bad news. This traumatic incident remains forever on my mind. I see it as a clear message that clinicians in all settings need training on breaking bad news to patients and their families.

25

My Work as a Palliative Care Nurse and Community Volunteer Coordinator at Mobile Hospice Mbarara (Hospice)

Betty Bifabusa

I joined Hospice Africa Uganda (HAU), of which MHM is one of three sites, in April 2007 from a curative hospital where I had worked for 13 years.

Understanding palliative care took me some time before I joined HAU; at the training school we were never taught about palliative care during our training.

Once I learned a little about palliative care, I was very excited to get this job, though my knowledge was just beginning. Before starting the job, I was told to first come to Mbarara and spend a week working with the team to understand the nature of work and the place itself. It was a tough time because I had not yet resigned officially from the hospital where I was working. I had to find a way to secure all the five days away from duty since my leave was not yet due.

Indeed, God was on my side because I was able to make it to Mbarara successfully. You can imagine the prayers at that time when looking for a new job. People I knew tried to discourage me and even scare me that any time I can be sent away from Hospice, but in my heart, I was firm about my decision. I wanted a change and wanted to learn new things; I was especially interested to know more about palliative care.

Finally, I arrived in Mbarara and on 2 April reported at Hospice to start working. What a warm welcome I received right from the gate. The Hospice team gathered in the conference hall for prayers and all other communications that morning – and every morning, I soon learned. I was introduced to the team members by the Health Services Coordinator (HSC). She took me around the place for orientation and I was assigned a mentor. Always I worked with a senior person in patient management. I successfully finished the probation and was confirmed for a permanent job in clinical care.

Next, I was sent for the training in palliative care (DCPC) which I completed successfully, acquiring more knowledge and skills in providing palliative care. Life at Hospice continued to improve for me and in 2009 I was chosen to be the Community Volunteers Coordinator.

At first I had some fears, especially with the language I would speak to these people in the community, as they speak Runyakore, which was new to me. I remember the HSC and Clinical Director that time told me when I was worried about the language that 'God will always give me the words to speak to his people.' This work exposed me to all the opportunities with my job. I got all the necessary support towards the new opportunities this work presented and at the end of the day I enjoyed it. Being the Community Volunteers Coordinator has since become a rewarding part of my life at Hospice.

Voluntary work is a gift from God; not everybody chooses to give of themselves as the CVWs do. CVWs have a great impact in bringing palliative care service close to the people. They can greatly improve the lives and well-being of patients with life-threatening illnesses and their families since they are looked at as caring colleagues and friends from within the community.

From the beginning, I was inspired by how the CVWs were so committed to support people in their communities in need of palliative care. Despite **no** payment, these people have love for the patients they care for till the time they pass on. Volunteers share their genuine love and care with patients and families and give all possible support for the challenges they face.

Even after someone passes on, they help us find ways forward, finding schools and homes for orphans, such as one young boy placed at the highly regarded Watoto School, children who receive schooling through HAU's Give a Chance project, and an abandoned/neglected child taken in by the Charity Sisters of Mother Teresa at Namugongo. Among the other tasks the CVWs carry out is arranging for the required documents from the district officials at no cost. Thanks to the CVWs' commitment, life for these children has improved and they can see light in their future.

CVWs taught me the Runyankore language and their culture. Through them I've gotten to know the community at large and been able to network with other organizations. For my support visits and supervision, we have always met at health facilities in the CVWs' communities. This enabled me to get to know other health workers, Village Health Teams (VHTs) and make local friends, hence increasing advocacy for palliative care.

This role has taught me to appreciate that knowledge is power; the CVWs have always had confidence in providing palliative Care from the training I provide at their ongoing updates. I also learnt that you do not need to have so much in the way of medical supplies or equipment with you to help someone; the only important thing you need is **LOVE.**

I treasure the CVWs for their commitment towards the work and thank the HAU management for motivating the CVWs to do their work despite reduced funding in recent years. Some of them are so self-motivated that even in this era of Covid-19, with all the risks of caring for people, and without the usual tools like patient care kits containing basic hygiene items, they continue to refer patients and visit them at home.

Hospice has helped me to grow in terms of work, good experience and learning the ethos of caring for patients and their families through the multi-disciplinary practice of palliative care.

Thank you, Dr Anne for the VISION which became a reality.

26

Ensuring Patients Enjoy a Hospitable Environment at Hospice Africa Uganda

Vicky Amazo

My name is Vicky Amazo and I serve as a General Assistant at HAU. I come from Arua district in the West Nile region of Uganda. When I was ten years old, I had a profound experience. One morning while I was sweeping the compound at home, I found myself crying out to the Lord. I prayed that God gives me a job when I grow up so that I could be able to pay school fees for my sisters. Our family was struggling to meet the costs of education for me and my siblings.

Although at that tender age I wanted with all my heart to become a nun, this was not to become the reality. I got married and then in 1995 when I was in my early 20s my husband, Daniel Amazo, left for Kampala, nearly 500 kilometres away, in search of a job. He had a dream of a better future for me and his family. He was a skilled gardener and HAU was quick to deploy his skills to tend the lawn and mind the flowers in the gardens surrounding the Hospice.

Hospice's founder, Dr Anne Merriman, soon enquired about Daniel's family and requested him to bring his wife to stay with him. This was the start of my 25-year journey with Hospice and Palliative Care. My husband, now deceased (may he rest in eternal peace), was my gate-pass into HAU, an organization I have grown to love because of the great mission they have for the suffering patient.

At HAU, the patient is the centre of the love and attention of not just the clinical team but all of us who work there. My first posting was as a General Assistant, and my goal became to ensure that wherever I cleaned not just looked great but sparkled. Some of the patients who come to Hospice are very sick and are feeling very low in their spirits. It, therefore, makes a lot of difference how they are welcomed and whether or not they are received and cared for in a clean, safe, and comfortable environment. I have always tried my best to see to it that the patient who walks into Hospice at dawn finds a clean and organized atmosphere.

Over the years I have worked at several jobs in the Hospice. When I worked in the kitchen, I endeavoured to prepare the food early so that the patients and the Hospice team would have a hot, nutritious meal ready for their lunch. Later on, I worked as a housekeeper in Fazal House. It served as a students' residence and welcomed many guests when academic semesters were not in session. Hospitality is at the heart of the Hospice philosophy and it has always been important to me that the guests who came to Fazal House felt that they were at home while away from their real homes.

I also worked for a brief period in the Morphine Production Unit. Hospice manufactures morphine but even before that process gets underway the pharmaceutical plant where the opioid is reconstituted must be extremely clean so that the medicine we manufacture is of the highest quality and acceptable for use by all who need pain relief in Uganda.

Today I am 50 years old or young, whichever way you look at it, and I continue to offer my services to the palliative care world. My attention these days is around patients and the ambiance they must find at HAU in Kampala so that they enjoy the care the nurses give them. I ensure patients are in a clean lounge and as they wait to see a clinician, I check to see that they have a cup of hot tea. I assist those who need to go to commodes, and I help families navigate from one room to another if they require assistance. I am always happy to give a glass of water to a patient who wants to swallow their first doses of medicine while still within the outpatients' rooms.

Although I never became a nun, I have found met my desire to serve those who are suffering, and I feel fulfilled in my work.

27

Necessity Is the Mother of Invention

COVID-19-inspired Innovations for Training Health Professionals in Africa

Eddie Mwebesa

For 14 years HAU has conducted the Palliative Care Initiators courses to train health professionals from throughout Africa, mostly doctors, pharmacists, nurses, social workers, and allied professionals, to initiate affordable and culturally appropriate Palliative Care Services in their own countries, and to be advocates and/or leaders for the specialty … but then abruptly came COVID-19, a word which did not exist until the last quarter of 2019! The coronavirus pandemic turned the world upside down, interrupting nearly all sectors of life, from tourism travel, and from the economy to education!

In 2019 while the grim reaper took many lives and air travel ground to a halt, the globe was so preoccupied with how to stop the many deaths, how to care for those who were severely ill, and how to prevent the infection from spreading that it was simply impossible to conduct the Initiators courses. Traditionally these courses involved travel to Uganda for five weeks with in-class didactic programs and then placements where students shadow

HAU's multidisciplinary teams at outpatient clinics and bedside teaching at patients' homes.

The World Health Organization highlights the central role of education and training of health professionals in its public health approach to palliative care, in order to meet the need to extend care to the multitudes suffering globally. With no courses possible due to travel restrictions and lockdowns to control the spread of the coronavirus yet, we knew many professionals who wanted to get palliative care training but the situation was 'business as abnormal'. HAU's Department of International Programmes (IP) innovatively restructured a previously in-person training program to become an online course with a placement session.

E-Learning is a modern approach to flexible studying which conveniently allows course attendance while participants are continuing to work and can circumvent restrictions on travel. The course promotes wide access to palliative care resources and life-long learning. New buzzwords like Zoom and Microsoft Teams were flying around, and it became clear very quickly that HAU had to embrace technology and use it to our advantage in this digital age. The IP team, therefore, underwent intensive training in 2020 and prepared to launch the new course in 2021.

To deliver what used to be a three week in-class teacher-student session, an online section was developed. It is now conducted over three months and deploys Moodle, an interactive, internet-based, virtual learning platform. Weekly mini lectures are held to increase real-time interaction with facilitators and course participants.

The placement presented a particular challenge because it is nearly impossible to substitute bedside teaching with technological alternatives. Clinical placement is therefore still necessary. This is a three-week long practicum in Uganda that comprises two weeks of experiential learning with the Hospice multi-disciplinary teams. During the placement, participants have mobile rounds with visits to patients in their homes, hands-on bedside teaching, observe morphine production, visit a hospital service and partners in palliative care, and then a one-week Training-of-Trainers programme to consolidate teaching and mentoring skills.

Necessity is indeed the mother of invention and HAU is beginning to reap the fruits of their innovations. The first online Anglophone Initiators Course was conducted in 2021 and completed by 31 participants with a Certificate of Online Attendance. Nine came for the first placement in May. Unfortunately, due to COVID-19 surges in several African countries, including Uganda, the second placement cohort had only two participants. All 11 received a Certificate of Completion of the course after their placement. The participants reported in their feedback that they found the course extremely beneficial and all 11 who attended the placement developed detailed Action Plans for commencing or advancing Palliative care in their organizations, hospitals, or countries. As alumni of our courses, they are included in the HAU official register, which we share with countries' central health authorities, as Palliative Care resource persons in their countries.

Finally, more fruits of the innovations are coming up! The first *online* Francophone course started on 30 August 2021. It followed a structure similar to its Anglophone counterpart. HAU has also received a request from a training institution in Southern Africa that is keen to adopt the innovations we instituted.

28

How Covid-19 Impacted Palliative Care

Martha Rabwoni

The global Covid-19 pandemic has had a devastating impact on patient care, and this impact has too 'metastasized' to cancer and chronic non-cancer patients on, and/or in need of palliative care. The enforcement of curfews and lockdown, coupled with temporary suspension of private and public transport to curb the spread of the virus has presented practical transport challenges to patients and their carers. In fact, initially at Hospice we adjusted the work schedules such that only one clinician per day was to be seeing patients; we presumed very few patients would be coming to the clinic given the transport challenges. Nonetheless, cancer pain is unbearable without medications to relieve the patient's pain, and in no time at all the one clinician overwhelmed by patients' numbers who needed palliative care.

So, one would wonder, how did patients manage to make it to the Hospice clinic amidst the odds of transport? The phone became a very useful tool in keeping communication flow between the Hospice team and patients, and their family carers. Most of our patients at Hospice come from very far and are out of the catchment area. Patients/family would call and we would advise them to get the passes to come to Hospice from their Local Council leadership. Then, they would get the movement pass from the RDCs. Of course, it was not easy, but some managed to navigate the bureaucratic and tiresome process and got the movement passes.

Agonizingly, some of our patients walked as far as 40 km to come and pick their medicines! Whilst some, especially the very frail and sick patients unable to sit on boda bodas, sent boda boda men to come and pick their treatment but still we needed to know the condition of the patient. The phone came into use again. Whenever the boda boda man would arrive at the clinic with or without the patient's medication chart, we would retrieve their case notes, call the patient and talk to them and try getting their condition and feelings in detail, and then we would count the medicines and send them via boda boda.

It has not been easy but doable. Patients' confidentiality was an issue because sometimes we had to ask what exactly the patient is complaining of, while they also had to share the details of their illnesses to the authorities to get travel passes. On some occasions, the boda man or family carer would arrive when the patient's phone was unreachable due to network connectivity issues or the battery being off. So, the boda man would himself tell you the patient's condition; others had no idea about the patient's condition. Sometimes, we had to call a neighbour, who would talk to the patient, or take the phone to the patient so the clinician eventually got to understand the patient's condition.

Financial constraints cannot fail to feature in the equation, given that majority of our patients are needy. Again, many come from very far and had to pay boda men who charge them as much as between double to thrice the normal cost to come pick their medicines. New patients referred from the referral hospital and other facilities would also come for care. These patients came from very far and were brought by ambulance and you would think the ambulance is free! Still the patients would pay for fuel, and sometimes allowance for the driver.

Here's an example of just one case of how getting care for patients is complicated in the time of Covid-19.

'Simon' was a man aged 68, HIV positive with advanced head and neck tumour. He had been a builder all his life yet had never built a house for himself. He had 10 children with two different women, of whom one died. Of his eight girls and two boys, both boys and four girls died.

Simon became very sick and was taken to several hospitals. The histology results confirmed squamous cell carcinoma, poorly differentiated keratinizing type involving skeletal muscles. While the plan was for him to get chemotherapy from Uganda Cancer Institute (UCI), he ran out of money. He was taken back home in terrible pain and unable to eat.

The landlord demanded his rent, so the neighbour called his uncle in Mbarara and said that the man had died they should go and pick the dead body. When the uncle arrived, he found Simon breathing and took him into his home where a Hospice-trained community volunteer worker (CVW) was called to see Simon, who he referred to Hospice.

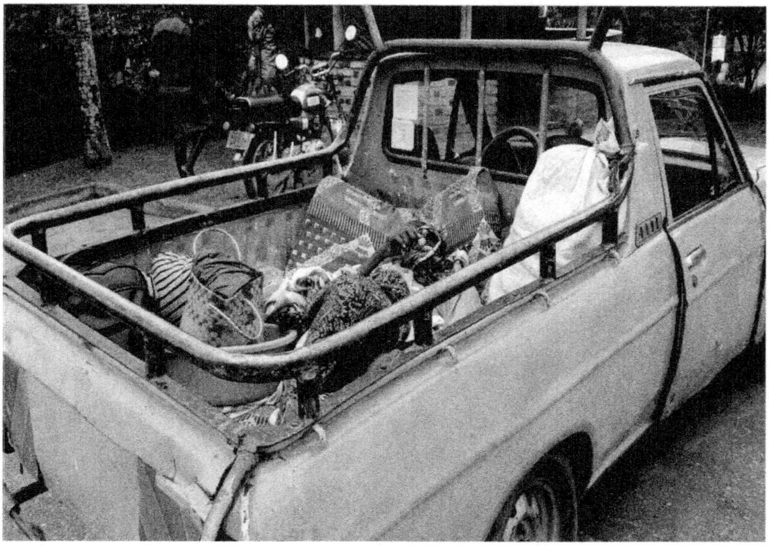

Photo 34 The pick-up car

Now the challenge was how to get the patient to Hospice. The uncle asked his friend who had a pick-up to give them a ride to Mbarara. The owner of the pick-up refused as he feared his car being impounded if they found there a person without a travel pass. The uncle of the patient insisted that his friend's car would be protected.

To beat the security curfew patrols, they started out at 5:30 am. No sooner had they reached the main road then they noticed the police were stopping every moving vehicle. The driver parked the car at a distance and ran away into hiding. Then the uncle had to think quickly; he put up his hand and told the police that they have a patient who is very sick and the car has run out of fuel and someone has gone to get fuel.

When the policeman glanced at the patient, he replied 'please be quick and take the patient.' So, the uncle called the driver on phone to come out of hiding and continue with the journey. Regrettably, the police demanded the only five thousand shillings they had on themselves, reported as 'for tea'.

The patient was truly very sick, in severe pain, dehydrated and could not swallow anything. We put him on a drip and gave him some morphine and he was able to utter a few words of thanks to the team. The uncle was so confused that he asked if there was any medicine which could revive the patient back to normal. He was given counselling on end-of life-care; the driver then drove the patient back home because if he died in hospital, it would be another hassle to take the body home. The patient died within a week, pain-free in the comfort of his uncle's home.

Indeed, in hard and unprecedented times like this Covid-19 pandemic, the vulnerable become more vulnerable and their suffering is amplified. Fortunately, with creativity, innovation, quick thinking and empathy, this suffering can be mitigated.

29

How Sylvia Came to Hospice Africa Uganda

Sylvia Dive

I wrote this story because every time I meet someone new at Hospice, the same question is asked: how did you come to be in Uganda? So I felt the need to put down something.

It was late 2008 when my aunt fell sick. I had finished my third year degree in Congo. My home area was torn apart by war, but my school district was safe.

My family and I agreed when I finished my nursing training that I should go to Uganda for a break as part of my after-studies adventure and to visit my dear aunt. However, after several expensive check-ups, my aunt's bone marrow test revealed a cancer called multiple myeloma. It was very sad! Indeed I cried. At first, her husband kept the results to himself, can you imagine!

With my little knowledge of medicine, I suspected that something serious was going on. As a matter of fact, I listed all the symptoms and signs of the disease that I had been seeing in my aunt. I sat down at the computer to find out; it took me time, for I was the main carer and to some extent I wasn't familiar with searching on the computer.

Two months later, her condition worsened. Her husband remained silent. If I knew how to break the bad news, I would have told my aunt myself. By that time, I had read all about multiple myeloma.

I continued grieving alone. Every time I entered her room my eyes were red. No one realized the cause of my sadness, but one evening my aunt asked me, 'Why are your eyes red?' I replied that I had been lighting the fire.

'That's not true,' she replied and added, 'Life is a journey, I am about to complete mine; my children are young, please wherever you will be, don't forget your cousins.'

I burst into tears. Indeed, she was right. Forty-two years of age. A mother of five children. The two older ones were sitting for S6 exams in boarding school. Their father didn't even want them to come home because their mother's health would affect them. Still the eldest would run from school in deep sorrow to see her mother in her wheelchair.

Her husband finally broke the bad news to the family when she was close to death, and then everybody in the family was angry with him. It distressed me and the rest of the family that he chose to keep silent, and I believe that has led to hatred among them. Normally the patient's beloved wants to see and care for their patient up to the end. It is a healing for them; once they know the patient's condition they prefer to pour out their love and effort to the patient and be near the patient. Many would have travelled from Congo to say their last words. She was in a coma, and to make it worse she was the most supportive and caring woman in the family.

One month after her death, her second youngest daughter (11 years old), who was still in P6 and used to be very close to her mother, suddenly said, 'I wish you had explained my mother's condition; I had many things to tell her.' We all kept quiet. Children are like mature people. May her soul rest in eternal peace, Amen.

Patients know their bodies better than we do. Although the husband kept the diagnosis for himself, still the aunty knew everything. We shouldn't deceive ourselves. We should respect patient autonomy and integrity, for it is their right, and it reduces the family's expectations for recovery. Telling the truth helps the family and patient to have realistic expectations and to begin to get used to the idea that their loved one is dying.

Eventually she died peacefully on 26 December 2008, under Hospice care after experiencing all the symptoms I had read on the internet. Up until today caring for a similar case is extremely upsetting, so I always refer it to my colleagues and that is the beauty of working as a team.

Caring for my aunt aroused my love and compassion for those who are dying. I asked Nurse Florence from Hospice if she could take me as a volunteer. She said yes and that was great news for me. She was a very courageous nurse. She was the main nurse who cared for my aunt up to the end. Even if we called at night, she would respond.

Such care really surprised the whole family because we were foreigners in Uganda, and there was a big language barrier. The care boosted my desire and energy to work in Hospice, and Florence advised me to write a distinct CV. I couldn't speak English or construct a phrase; so that advice discouraged me. Despite my limits in writing and reading English, one Tuesday I brought my CV to the volunteer coordinator, Ms Catherine. She gave me the form to fill in and asked me to choose the programmes. I preferred Tuesday and Thursday, since I was still taking care of my cousins. I returned home and the following day, I was in Hospice. What a beautiful team to work with!

There was a team leader, Nurse Charlotte, who would make fun of me because I couldn't express myself in English well, but that was not an issue for me. I was so focused on understanding the clinical skill in palliative care.

One Thursday I sat beside an old and well-dressed beautiful woman in the case conference. She asked me one question; I couldn't get what she was saying. First of all, she was speaking faster, with an English accent. Secondly she asked me who I was. Immediately she realized that my accent was different. She continued 'Where are you from?' I replied quietly, 'From Congo.' She went on to ask me in which department I was volunteering. I replied, 'Clinical Department.' My answers were short.

Finally, some days later, she started looking for me at Hospice. Unfortunately, she had forgotten my name and all other details. She kept looking for me as a Nigerian lady; no one was helping her and there were many volunteers at

Hospice as well. We could meet in the compound but still I dodged her out of fear.

Surprisingly, one day we met face to face, and she shouted, 'Here she is!' Oh! I got scared. But being a very wise woman, she was able to read my fear; she held my hand. This was Dr Anne. Peacefully we walked into her office, and she served me a cup of tea and a biscuit, which reduced my anxiety. Amazingly, she called the very nurse Florence who was the health services coordinator and indeed she knew me better than others.

My heartbeat increased and I sweated everywhere. We had a brief interview, and she took my photo. Meanwhile, I had a lot of fear because my visa had expired. My aunt's condition required lots of money. However, aunt's husband promised to pay the visa later when we had settled a bit after her loss. We separated, and she told me to let her know if I was to leave Uganda. Of course, I went back to Congo. I had a fiancé who couldn't wait, so he had got another woman. It was really a dilemma for me because I had to care for my aunty. It really disturbed me psychologically when I reached Congo, so as soon as I returned to Uganda I wrote to Dr Anne.

I continued with my volunteer work. One morning her personal secretary called me to pass on Dr Anne's message that she had got a sponsor for me and that I should be ready to start an initiator course for five weeks. As soon as I got an email from my sponsor, Mrs Jim Bennett, asking me to write briefly how I came to Uganda and a history of my family and enclose my photo. I was so eager and impatient to start the course and I performed well, because my communication skills had improved a bit.

Hospice has three different sites. One of the sites was lacking a nurse, so I was sent to support as a locum. Unfortunately, I wasn't qualified to work without the consent of the Nursing Council and work permit, because I am a foreigner. I was called back for interview and internship in the National Referral Hospital, Mulago and finally got my registration from the Nursing Council; I scored 81%.

Soon after I became Hospice staff. I was quite happy and afterwards enrolled for long clinical diploma course, sponsored by Hospice Africa France, led by Mr Jim Bennett. I graduated in February 2014 and did several short courses in palliative care after.

I would like to express my sincere gratitude to Professor Anne, Jim, and Florence. They made me who I am; I got a lot of opportunities that I wouldn't otherwise have had. I can't mention all, but it has shaped my life history.

I met another boyfriend at Hospice while at his pastoral duties; both of us are Congolese from different regions. I am living with him and have one child.

I managed to complete the Master's in Public Health with the help of Hospice Africa (HA) Uganda and HA France, I hope to graduate in 2023 and proceed for other levels.

Language has been a barrier. It is hard to learn a second language fluently, such as English but when you love what you are doing the challenge become a learning point and not a discouragement. At school my teachers called me a

Franco-English speaker because I think in French and I agree with them. Our executive director, Dr Doreen, keeps saying: '*Love what you do and keep going.*'

I now coordinate the training for Francophone countries from Hospice, under International Programmes (IP). It was a privilege to work closely for ten years with the founder of Hospice Africa Uganda and I have learned a lot. Palliative care has changed me in different ways.

I have loved every step of the way.

30

Dr Anne Merriman's Palliative Care Vision

A Legacy of Empathy and Faith

Naomi Nasasira

My first encounter with Hospice Africa Uganda (HAU) was with the founder, Dr Anne Merriman in January 1994 in Kampala. My late father had gone through treatment of the cancer of the oesophagus about two or three months earlier in the UK. Dr Anne was new in Uganda, and I got information about her from the Cancer Institute of Mulago Hospital where I had gone looking for help for him. He had contacted a bad cough most likely from guests who were then flocking his home to welcome him back after months of absence. His immunity was very low following Radiotherapy and Chemotherapy treatment. He was also not young, about 88 years then.

Dr Anne's contacts, telephone number, and a map to her residence were on a piece of paper of the Cancer Institute's reception noticeboard. It was a Saturday evening and I had been moving around hospitals and clinics looking for help most of the day. The Cancer Institute was the scariest part of the hospital to think of visiting. I was desperate and ready to go anywhere and everywhere for my father.

From her landline Dr Anne guided me to her home, listened to my problem and gave my father treatment that evening. She visited him the following day after her church service and she took him on as her patient from that day and together with her team supported him until he passed in June 1999 a period of about five and a half years. Dr Anne and the team cared for my father. My family was deeply touched. My mother who passed on a few months ago benefitted from the same HAU team in managing her old age illnesses. Who would not be grateful! My family is just a sample representing many families that have tasted the care of HAU.

Dr Anne approached a few of us to be volunteers and I served on the HAU first Advisory Committee in 1994. I was Vice to the late Mr Kateregga who served as the chairman. She encouraged me to take on a leadership role even though at the time I did not think I would be able to do it. I later served on the Board of Directors and eventually retired from the Board in 2008. I have since served in other areas of HAU and I remain a life member.

The role played by HA in Uganda as a model and in the many African countries is noble, to say the least. Now people in these African countries where HA is operating know that every life matters to the end. They have learnt and tested pain control and providing quality life to patients, even those who are not health workers have acquired skills in managing the sick.

The good gospel of caring has spread in many corners of our countries. The status of nurses in Uganda has changed. A HAU nurse is not an ordinary nurse. They are confident and knowledgeable and ably treat terminally ill patients. They are authorities, in their own right, and respected more than before. They are also kind, approachable, and treat patients with care and respect. This is not what a Ugandan nurse was in the past.

The Institute of Palliative Care which started as a training department in HAU is now a tertiary institution awarding certificates, diplomas and degrees in palliative care. This is one amazing dream come true. Dr Anne's vision has not only succeeded in Uganda but beyond to many countries of Africa.

Dr Anne has great empathy with people but more so with people in disadvantaged positions. She is always looking for how to help those in need, how to relieve the pain, the suffering, and for where it could be better for a human being. She recently told me that she feels bad that she will leave this world when Ugandan children are still being beaten in schools.

Dr Anne taught people to be kind and to care for the sick, to provide for the needy and to share with those who have less. We undertook many activities to create awareness and to fundraise for HAU. These included charity walks, flea markets, retreats, workshops to name but a few. All in the effort to raise money to support people in need. She preached love and practised love. Her family in Munyonyo is the best testament of Jaja's love.

Dr Anne mobilized funding for Hospice Africa (HA), thanks to the many donors who trusted her with their funds and have made it possible for an organization that started in a small room to become a serious entity with blocks of buildings of its own. All funded by Anne's contacts. Thanks to all those who have contributed in many ways to what HAU is today. Looking as far back as 1994 I can only say that truly 'faith moves mountains'. Anne's faith created HA.

A legacy of empathy and faith is my description of Dr Anne's contribution to mankind in the African part of the globe. Thank you, Anne, and thank you to all who have joined her to make HA what it is.

The young team currently managing HAU is doing a fantastic job. They are a source of survival and continuity for our Hospice and deserve our support to succeed. Together we will succeed.

May God our Heavenly father bless each one of us with the will to give a hand.

Index

Page numbers in bold refer to photographs and photo captions

Printed in Great Britain
by Amazon

23196587R00089